Managing Stress in Music Education

Managing Stress in Music Education presents research, theory, possible pitfalls, and strategies for music teachers looking to navigate the challenging climate of potential stressors.

Covering a wide range of topics such as sleep, physical movement, nutrition, happiness, gratitude, and mindfulness, this book offers music educators the tools to thrive in a work environment that can often lead to stress and burnout. Readers will examine vignettes of challenged and successful music teachers, and consider new techniques and classic reminders for a healthy enjoyment of work and life.

Grounded in research and written in an accessible and concise manner, *Managing Stress in Music Education* is an excellent addition to any music teacher's bookshelf.

H. Christian Bernhard II is Professor of Music at the State University of New York at Fredonia.

Routledge New Directions in Music Education Series
Series Editor: Clint Randles

The Routledge New Directions in Music Education Series consists of concise monographs that attempt to bring more of the wide world of music, education, and society into the discourse in music education.

Eco-Literate Music Pedagogy
Daniel J. Shevock

The Music Profiles Learning Project
Let's Take This Outside
Radio Cremata, Gareth Dylan Smith, Joseph Michael Pignato, and Bryan Powell

A Different Paradigm in Music Education
Re-examining the Profession
David A. Williams

Eudaimonia
Perspectives for Music Learning
Edited by Gareth Dylan Smith and Marissa Silverman

Managing Stress in Music Education
Routes to Wellness and Vitality
H. Christian Bernhard II

Managing Stress in Music Education
Routes to Wellness and Vitality

H. Christian Bernhard II

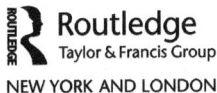
NEW YORK AND LONDON

First published 2021
by Routledge
605 Third Avenue, New York, NY 10017

and by Routledge
2 Park Square, Milton Park, Abingdon, Oxon OX14 4RN

First issued in paperback 2022

Routledge is an imprint of the Taylor & Francis Group, an informa business

© 2021 Taylor & Francis

The right of H. Christian Bernhard II to be identified as author of this work has been asserted by him in accordance with sections 77 and 78 of the Copyright, Designs and Patents Act 1988.

All rights reserved. No part of this book may be reprinted or reproduced or utilised in any form or by any electronic, mechanical, or other means, now known or hereafter invented, including photocopying and recording, or in any information storage or retrieval system, without permission in writing from the publishers.

Trademark notice: Product or corporate names may be trademarks or registered trademarks, and are used only for identification and explanation without intent to infringe.

Publisher's Note
The publisher has gone to great lengths to ensure the quality of this reprint but points out that some imperfections in the original copies may be apparent.

Library of Congress Cataloging-in-Publication Data
Names: Bernhard, H. Christian, II, author.
Title: Managing stress in music education / H. Christian Bernhard II.
Description: New York: Routledge, 2020. |
Series: Routledge new directions in music education series |
Includes bibliographical references and index.
Identifiers: LCCN 2020020035 (print) | LCCN 2020020036 (ebook) |
ISBN 9780367434540 (hardback) | ISBN 9781003003366 (ebook)
Subjects: LCSH: Music teachers–Job stress. | Stress management.
Classification: LCC MT1.B544 M36 2020 (print) |
LCC MT1.B544 (ebook) | DDC 780.71–dc23
LC record available at https://lccn.loc.gov/2020020035
LC ebook record available at https://lccn.loc.gov/2020020036

ISBN: 978-0-367-56364-6 (pbk)
ISBN: 978-0-367-43454-0 (hbk)
ISBN: 978-1-003-00336-6 (ebk)

DOI: 10.4324/9781003003366

Typeset in Times New Roman
by Newgen Publishing UK

In loving memory of my mother, Cynthia Petersen Bernhard

Contents

Series Editor Foreword   viii

1 Routes   1
2 Sleep   8
3 Physical Movement   19
4 Nutrition   29
5 Gratitude   40
6 Happiness   51
7 Mindfulness   63
8 Roots   75

Index   85

Series Editor Foreword

Routledge New Directions in Music Education Series consists of concise monographs that attempt to bring more of the wide world of music, education, and society – and all of the conceptualizations and pragmatic implications that come with that world – into the discourse in music education. It is about discovering and uncovering big ideas for the profession, criticizing our long held assumptions, suggesting new courses of action, and putting ideas into motion for the prosperity of future generations of music makers, teachers of music, researchers, scholars, and society.

Clint Randles, Series Editor

1 Routes

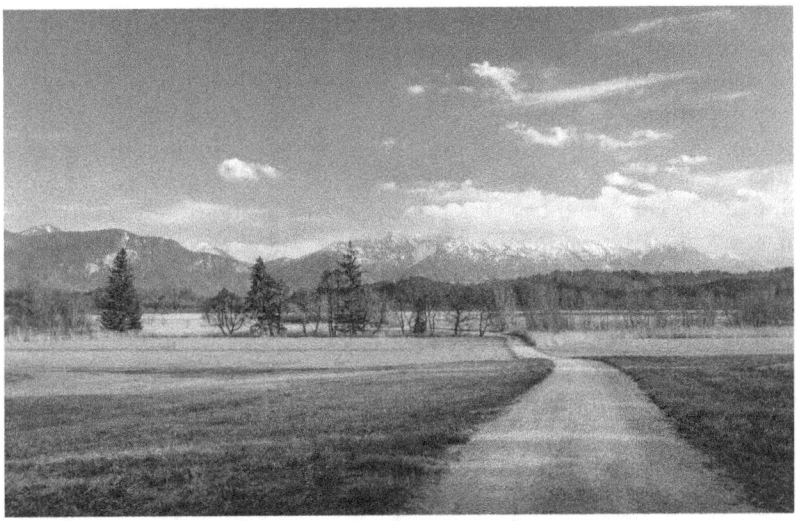

Figure 1.1 Routes
Source: Mario Dobelman, Unsplash, https://unsplash.com/

Teaching music can be a rewarding, yet stressful, profession. While many music educators are drawn to teaching by a passion for creative music making and inspiring others to learn, challenges such as classroom management, administrative tasks, and political mandates can cause stress, and if unchecked, burnout. These issues are particularly acute for current music teachers, as they respond to initiatives such as Common Core Standards in English Language Arts and Math, increasing scrutiny regarding annual evaluation, and changes in certification requirements such as Pearson's Teacher Performance Assessment (edTPA), while simultaneously facing fiscal challenges that have resulted in elimination of teaching positions and shifts in responsibilities (e.g., National Association for Music Education, 2015).

The majority of this book was written during the final months of 2019, but this opening chapter is being completed as the global pandemic of COVID-19 consumes public thought and attention. Music teachers are moving to distance education platforms such as Google Classroom, and struggling to replicate traditional performance opportunities for their students and audience members. Pre-service teachers are completing degree requirements using virtual programs such as Zoom, and are wondering whether mandated field experiences and certification exams will be waived, or whether jobs will even be available at the other end of the process. All of these challenges on top of daily newsfeeds, both real and fake, that people are sick and dying, and that the economy is suffering. Never before has attention to stress been so very important.

Gold and Roth (2003) defined stress as "a condition of disequilibrium within the intellectual, emotional, and physical state of the individual; it is generated by one's perceptions of a situation, which result in physical and emotional reactions." (p. 17). They stated that most teachers experience moderate levels of stress on a fairly regular basis, and that good stress, or "eustress," can actually be a positive component of teaching. However, when perceptions spin out of control, or when challenges become too intense, negative stress, or "distress," can lead to burnout. According to Vandenberghe and Huberman (1999), burnout is "a crisis of overworked and disillusioned human service workers" (p. 1). This syndrome has been extended to members of the teaching profession and has been categorized into three distinct components; emotional exhaustion, depersonalization, and reduced personal accomplishment (Maslach, Jackson, & Leiter, 1996).

Byrne (1999) conducted a review of research literature regarding teacher burnout to determine the contributions of background, organizational, and personality variables. Regarding background variables, she found that younger teachers tended to report higher levels of emotional exhaustion than older teachers and that high school teachers reported greater levels of overall burnout than elementary and middle school teachers. Regarding organizational variables, she found that role conflict, role ambiguity, work overload, and classroom climate contributed to teacher burnout. Finally, personality variables including locus of control and self-esteem were related to teacher burnout.

Other researchers have conducted studies specifically related to teachers of music. Conway, Micheel-Mays, and Micheel-Mays (2005) shared experiences of two early-career music teachers, and found that challenges included lack of time, exhaustion, feelings of isolation, need for validation, lack of job security, and need for personal reflection. Similarly, Sindberg and Lipscomb (2005) investigated professional isolation among 36 music teachers and found that, while differences were not observed based on school setting (urban, rural, or suburban), less experienced teachers reported more feelings of isolation than teachers with at least ten years of experience. They also found that many participants desired more contact with other teachers of music, and that, in some cases, isolation resulted in burnout and job resignation. Hedden (2005) conducted a longitudinal investigation of stress among 62 music educators. While she did not observe differences based on gender or school setting (urban or nonurban), she did find that participants indicated less stress after a seven-year period. Specifically, she found improvements in time management, work-related stressors, professional distress, and discipline and motivation, and suggested that teachers may be able to better manage stress as a result of maturation and teaching experience.

More recently, I compared perceived levels of burnout among 258 teachers by grade level taught, certification status, and music area (Bernhard, 2016). Participants who taught a combination of grade levels reported more severe levels of burnout than those who taught elementary, middle, or high school exclusively, beginning teachers reported more severe levels of burnout than more experienced teachers, and those who taught a combination of general, choral, and instrumental music reported more severe levels of burnout than their colleagues who taught general, choral, or instrumental music exclusively. Additionally, for combined subjects, moderate relationships were observed among burnout and hours per week of teaching, sleeping, relaxing, and working another job.

To combat music teacher stress and burnout, recent authors have recommended strategies including space for reflection and renewal (Tricarico, 2018), cognitive behavioral therapy (Herman & Reinke, 2015), and, ironically, even music therapy (Moffat, 2020). Herman and Reinke developed a model for coping with teacher stress in which they suggested awareness as an initial step. "Stress and stressors are neither good nor bad in themselves. What determines how they affect us, favorably or not, is how we interpret and respond to them" (p. 11). By monitoring thoughts and feelings, the authors suggested that teachers can manage resulting behaviors, mitigating personal problems and promoting effective school learning environments.

Similarly, the field of positive psychology has blossomed over the past two decades, and associated researchers have found that practices related to gratitude, happiness, and mindfulness can be helpful in alleviating and proactively managing teacher stress. McCullough, Emmons, and Tsang (2002) found gratitude to be positively related to optimism and life satisfaction, while negatively related to depression, anxiety, materialism, and envy. Emmons (2007) further documented that gratitude can enhance willpower, improve creativity, deepen spirituality, increase self-esteem, and enhance academic performance. Bono (2020) suggested that happiness – a combination of positive emotion, meaning, and engagement – should be considered as a fluid continuum instead of a binary on or off.

> At any given point, circumstances or conditions may be beyond our control. By asking what we can do to become *happier,* we place our attention on those aspects of life that *are* in our control, which ultimately can move us forward on the happiness continuum.
>
> (p. 10)

Srinivasan (2014) defined mindfulness as "energy we cultivate through kind, present-moment awareness" (p. 27). Kahn (2019) added that mindfulness involves a level of curiosity and non-judgement, observing thoughts and actions without assigning formal assessment. It involves recognition of the present, inhabiting the physical body and recognizing current surroundings.

From an even more organic perspective, human health depends on solid foundations of sleep, physical movement, and nutrition, and these variables are the focus of the following three chapters. If only one lifestyle change can be made in the immediate future, sleep is a pressing issue to address. "There does not seem to be one major organ within the body, or process within the brain, that isn't optimally enhanced by sleep" (Walker, 2018, p. 7). While the term "exercise" is sometimes considered as negative or pejorative, physical movement is a very normal and essential part of the human condition (e.g., Rath, 2013; Wachob, 2016). In addition to maintaining and improving muscle function, heart health, and immune systems, moving ourselves improves brain processing and emotional health (Ratey, 2008). Finally, practicing good nutrition can help to prevent heart attacks, diabetes, and cancer. It can also help to avoid stroke, osteoporosis, constipation, cataracts, and age-related memory loss (Willett & Skerrett, 2017).

Collectively, the purpose of this book is to present research, theory, and best practices related to sleep, physical movement, nutrition, gratitude, happiness, and mindfulness. While serious challenges should be addressed by professional medical providers, considering these six variables as routes to general health can help to create a mental and physical pathway to wellness and vitality. Although grounded in research, the writing style and concise nature of coverage of this book are intended to be digestible by busy music educators and college students. Vignettes of hypothetical, yet typical, music educators will further help to set a framework for both pre-service and in-service readers.

Summary

- Teaching can be a stressful occupation.
- Music teachers, in particular, are susceptible to burnout.
- Life stressors beyond music teaching add layers of further challenge.
- Create space for self-care.
- Consult medical professionals and consider therapeutic interventions.
- Embrace gratitude, happiness, and mindfulness (positive psychology).
- Embrace sleep, physical movement, and nutrition.

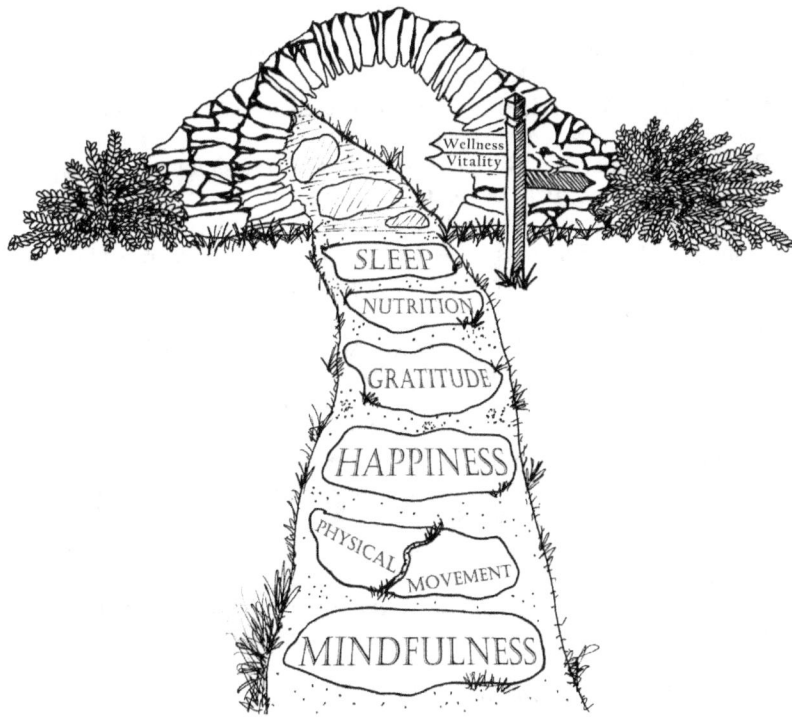

Figure 1.2 Zimmerman hand drawing 1
Source: Routes to Wellness and Vitality, Samantha Zimmerman.

References

Bernhard, H. C. (2016). Investigating burnout among elementary and secondary school music educators: A replication. *Contributions to Music Education, 41,* 145–156.

Bono, T. (2020). *Happiness 101: Simple secrets to smart living and well-being.* New York, NY: Grand Central.

Byrne, B. M. (1999). The nomological network of teacher burnout: A literature review and empirically validated model. In R. Vandenberghe & A. M. Huberman (Eds.), *Understanding and preventing teacher burnout: A sourcebook of international research and practice* (pp. 15–37). Cambridge: Cambridge College Press.

Conway, C. M., Micheel-Mays, L., & Micheel-Mays, C. (2005). A narrative study of student teaching and the first year of teaching: Common issues and struggles. *Bulletin of the Council for Research in Music Education, 165,* 65–77.

Emmons, R. A. (2007). *Thanks!: How practicing gratitude can make you happier.* New York, NY: Houghton Mifflin Harcourt Publications.

Gold, Y. & Roth, R. A. (2003). *Teachers managing stress and preventing burnout. The professional health solution.* New York, NY: Routledge.

Hedden, D. (2005). A study of stress and its manifestations among music educators. *Bulletin of the Council for Research in Music Education, 166,* 57–67.

Herman, K. C. & Reinke, W. M. (2015). *Stress management for teachers. A proactive guide.* New York, NY: Guilford Press.

Kahn, M. (2019). Mindfulness training. Retrieved June 1, 2019, from https://www.mindfulnesstrainingsrc.com/

Maslach, C., Jackson, S. E., & Leiter, M. P. (1996). *Maslach Burnout Inventory – Manual* (3rd ed.). Palo Alto, CA: College of California, Consulting Psychologists Press.

McCullough, M. E., Emmons, R. A., & Tsang, J. (2002). The grateful disposition: A conceptual and empirical topography. *Journal of Personality and Social Psychology, 82,* 112–127.

Moffat, L. (2020). *I love my job but it's killing me. The teacher's guide to conquering chronic stress and sickness.* New York, NY: Morgan James.

National Association for Music Education. (2015). *Teacher burnout is real: Signs and how to avoid it.* Retrieved May 21, 2015, from www.nafme.org/category/newsletter/orchestrating-success-newsletter

Ratey, J. J. (2008). *Spark: The revolutionary new science of exercise and the brain.* New York, NY: Little, Brown Spark.

Rath, T. (2013). *Eat, move, sleep: How small choices lead to big changes.* San Jose, CA: Missionday.

Sindberg, L. & Lipscomb, S. D. (2005). Professional isolation and the public school music teacher. *Bulletin of the Council for Research in Music Education, 166,* 43–56.

Srinivasan, M. (2014). *Teach, breathe, learn: Mindfulness in and out of the classroom.* Berkeley, CA: Parallax Press.

Tricarico, D. (2018). *Sanctuaries: Self-care secrets for stressed-out teachers.* San Diego, CA: Dave Burgess Consulting.

Vandenberghe, R., & Huberman, A. M. (1999). *Understanding and preventing teacher burnout: A sourcebook of international research and practice.* Cambridge: Cambridge College Press.

Wachob, J. (2016). *Wellth: How to build a life, not a résumé.* New York, NY: Harmony Books.

Walker, M. (2018). *Why we sleep: Unlocking the power of sleep and dreams.* New York, NY: Scribner.

Willett, W., & Skerrett, P. (2017). *Eat, drink and be healthy: The Harvard Medical School guide to healthy eating.* New York, NY: Simon & Schuster.

2 Sleep

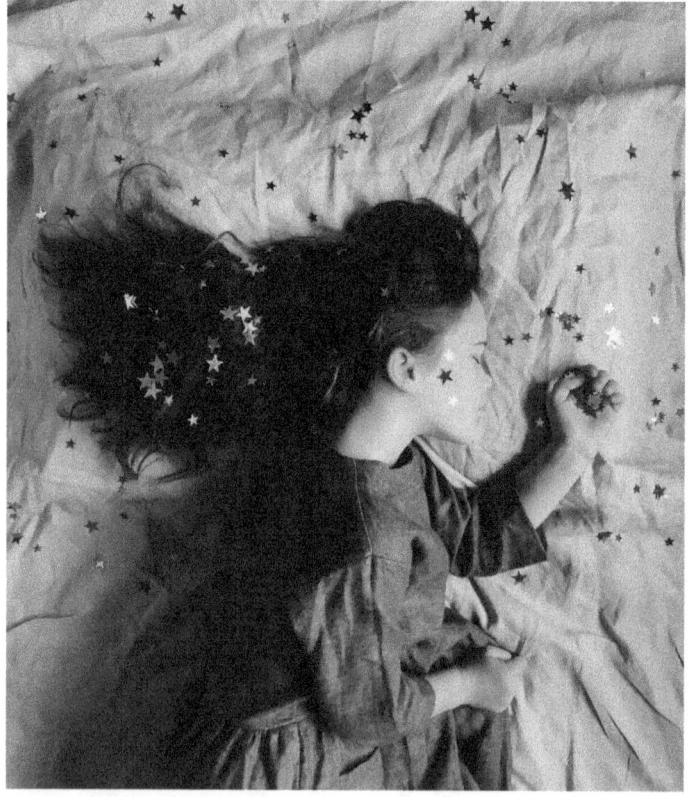

Figure 2.1 Sleep
Source: Annie Spratt, Unsplash, https://unsplash.com/

Zach feels frustrated as he struggles to keep his eyes open. Once again, he sits in the middle of his 9:00 a.m. music education methods class, feeling as though he could fall off his chair from exhaustion at any point. "I thought I slept better last night," Zach thinks to himself. "I made a point of getting in bed by 1:00 a.m. instead of staying awake until 2:00 or 3:00, like I normally do." But Zach is still suffering from severe sleep deprivation, averaging only five hours per night on a regular basis. Last night, he performed in a wind ensemble concert until 10:00, helped move percussion equipment until 10:45, played broomball with some friends until 11:30, consumed the better part of a whole pizza and a liter of soda until midnight, and crammed for an upcoming English exam, with interspersed checks of Twitter and Instagram, until crashing at 1:00 a.m. This morning, Zach slept through three alarms, abruptly waking ten minutes before class, skipping breakfast, and running to the music building. He likes the content of the current methods course, the professor, and his peers, but can only impatiently stare at the clock, praying that the 50-minute period will be over as soon as possible. He is unable to focus, and takes nothing from the morning session. Like many music education majors, Zach is struggling to balance music education, performance, and general education coursework, while also negotiating relationships with peers and living away from home for the first time. Without adjustments to sleep routines, his challenges will only multiply when student teaching and first-year assignments involve start times as early as 6:00 a.m.

According to the National Sleep Foundation (2019), 60 percent of American adults suffer from occasional sleep problems and over 40 million experience chronic sleep disorders, such as insomnia, sleep apnea, and narcolepsy. Furthermore, at least 40 percent of adults suffer from daytime sleepiness severe enough to interfere with work and other normal activities. Buysse (2014) suggested that sleep health can be measured on a ten-point scale, collecting zero–two points each for

> Satisfaction (are you satisfied with your sleep?), Alertness (do you stay awake all day?), Timing (are you asleep between 2:00 and 4:00 a.m.?), Efficiency (do you spend less than 30 minutes awake at night?), and Duration (do you sleep between 6 and 8 hours per night?).
>
> (p. 17B)

Problems sleeping often indicate underlying stress, and, when ignored, can lead to professional decline, deteriorating personal relationships, sickness, and even death (e.g., Lightman, 2018; Peterson, 2018; Rath, 2013; Shojai, 2016; Wachob, 2016; Walker, 2018). In fact, in a series of studies from the 1800s that would fortunately no longer pass animal rights protocol, researchers found that dogs who were purposefully deprived of sleep could not survive beyond a period of just a few days (Bentivoglio & Grassi-Zucconi, 1997). Furthermore, a report from the *New York Times* suggested that as little as six hours of sleep per night for a period of two weeks could produce similar states to that of being drunk (Jones, 2011), and "routinely sleeping less than six or seven hours a night demolishes your immune system, more than doubling your risk of cancer" (Walker, 2018, p. 3). While the following chapters addressing physical movement, nutrition, gratitude, happiness, and mindfulness are very important, sleep may trump all of them in terms of immediate importance. If only one lifestyle change can be made in the immediate future, sleep is a pressing issue to address. "There does not seem to be one major organ within the body, or process within the brain, that isn't optimally enhanced by sleep" (Walker, 2018, p. 7).

The challenge can be particularly acute for music teachers and their students, who not only belong to school systems starting early each morning, but often have before-school rehearsals or other activities, when sleep has not been fully completed, or after-school obligations that interfere with natural napping needs. Walker (2018) stated that there are two primary types of sleep personality; morning larks and night owls. Larks are genetically programmed to wake and thrive early, while owls have difficulty falling asleep until after midnight, and typically do not function optimally during morning hours. Music teachers who naturally lean toward owl tendencies might lobby for first period planning or study hall-type responsibilities, saving more intense rehearsals and other obligations for later in the day, or after school. Similarly, larks will tend to thrive in typical K-12 schedules, but could further enhance productivity by scheduling before-school rehearsals and early morning productivity (keeping in mind that many students, particularly middle and high school, may struggle early in the morning). Wahlstrom (2002) described the benefits of later starting times for high school students. She reported that seven high schools in the Minneapolis School District moved the beginning of school days from 7:15 a.m. to 8:40 a.m., and found improved student attendance, more alert students, and lower rates of student-reported depression. Walker (2018) supported these findings, stating "unnecessarily bankrupting the sleep of a teenager could make all the difference in the precarious tipping point between psychological wellness and lifelong psychiatric illness" (p. 309).

Healthy sleep involves both REM (rapid eye movement) and NREM periods (non-rapid eye movement). NREM sleep supports the storing of long-term memory, prunes neural networks, and typically involves relatively slow waves of brain activity. REM sleep, in contrast, features faster brain waves, builds neural networks, produces states of dream, and fosters processing of creativity and emotional regulation (Walker, 2018). "When we're exhausted, our brains can't help but focus on the negative. But when we get our eight hours, our brains reset and we are on a more even keel" (Barker, 2017, p. 229). Yoo, Gujar, Hu, Jolesz, and Walker (2007) studied the effects of sleep deprivation on the emotional responses of healthy adults between the ages of 18 and 30. The researchers assigned 26 participants to random groups of normal sleep and sleep deprivation (keeping those participants awake for 35 hours). They then gave participants 100 images to view, and recorded brain activity using functional magnetic resonance imaging (fMRI). Through scans of participants' amygdala, a key part of the brain responsible for processing emotion, the researchers found that sleep deprived participants had significantly more hyper and emotionally inappropriate responses to negative stimuli than participants who had slept normally. "It therefore seems that a night of sleep may 'reset' the correct brain reactivity to next-day emotional challenges by maintaining functional integrity of this amygdala circuit, and thus govern appropriate behavioral repertoires" (p. 878).

In addition to promoting cognitive and emotional growth, sound sleep can aid in development of motor skills, something of particular importance to musicians. Walker and Stickgold (2010) examined the effects of sleep on speed and accuracy of motor skills. They taught adult participants a set of left-handed number typing patterns on a computer keyboard. All of the participants had 12 minutes to practice the typing patterns and were then retested 12 hours later. Half of the participants were taught in the morning, were tested later that evening after no sleep, and showed no significant improvement in speed or accuracy. The other half of participants were taught during the evening, tested the following morning after a full night of sleep, and demonstrated a 20 percent gain in speed and 35 percent gain in accuracy. Even more impressive, the first group demonstrated similar improvements following a full night of sleep, with no further practice or instruction. Thus, musicians trying to improve motor skill performance might be wise to "sleep on it" instead of practicing endlessly at the expense of quality slumber.

Recommendations for Sound Sleep

While severe sleep challenges should be reported to a medical professional, researchers recommend several strategies for improving rest and renewal (e.g., National Sleep Foundation, 2019; Pang, 2018; Walker, 2018). A good starting point is keeping a consistent sleep schedule. This is usually a relatively easy task for K-12 music educators, who typically have the same work schedule each day, but can be challenging for music education majors, who often have very different class and rehearsal schedules on each day of a given week. Keeping a consistent schedule can also be difficult during weekends and holidays, when there is a temptation to sleep-in and stay up late. Instead, stick as close as possible to weekday schedules, while allowing a bit of flexibility for socializing and other enjoyable activities.

Naps can also be useful for afternoon renewal, but should be limited to approximately 30 minutes or less, as long and deep sleep can make it difficult to fall and stay asleep during regular night hours. When possible, some music teachers find it useful to take 15–20 minutes of alone time during a lunch period or at the end of a teaching day, perhaps lying on an exercise mat, or closing their eyes in a comfortable chair. Researchers have found that even a short nap can be effective in recharging mental batteries (Pang, 2018).

> The true pattern of biphasic sleep – for which there is anthropological, biological, and genetic evidence, and which remains measurable in all human beings to date – is one consisting of a longer bout of continuous sleep at night, followed by a shorter midafternoon nap.
>
> (Walker, 2018, p. 70)

Morning caffeine can be a tempting way to feel more alert. However, portion size should be monitored (Starbucks' "Venti" packs 20–24 ounces of liquid depending on whether it's served hot or cold) and caffeine consumption should cease at least eight hours before bedtime. Caffeine works to numb sleep receptors in the brain, which are sensitive to adenosine (Walker, 2018). Adenosine is a natural chemical that builds in the brain as the day progresses, encouraging feelings of sleepiness by the time night falls. However, if caffeine is still numbing the workings of adenosine, one can feel awake, only to crash miserably once the brain again senses adenosine. Even small amounts of caffeine still present hours after consumption can inhibit sleep quality.

In a comprehensive review of research literature, Clark and Landolt (2017) reported that, over the course of numerous studies, "caffeine typically prolonged sleep latency, reduced total sleep time and sleep efficiency, and worsened perceived sleep quality" (p. 70), particularly during slow-wave NREM sleep.

Alcohol and food consumption should also be limited close to bedtime. While both can induce feelings of sleepiness, they will disrupt rest throughout the night, negatively impacting quality of sleep (National Sleep Foundation, 2019). Ebrahim, Shapiro, Williams, and Fenwick (2013) conducted a review of literature regarding the impact of alcohol consumption on the sleep of healthy research participants. They reported that, while alcohol usually accelerates the transition from full wakefulness to sleep (sleep onset latency), it disrupts sleep quality, particularly during the second half of the night. During all parts of sleep, alcohol tends to disrupt patterns of REM sleep, the process that builds neural networks, produces states of dream, and fosters creativity and emotional regulation.

Keep the sleep environment cool and dark. "During sleep, our core body temperature dips, allowing us to slip into restorative REM and (NREM) slow-wave sleep" (Patz, 2019, p. 88). It may be tempting to crank up the heat, or use heavy blankets, but doing so can raise body temperature to the point that it becomes difficult to fall asleep or remain sleeping throughout the night. Even mattresses, pillows, and bedsheets can impact temperature levels, with the potential to disrupt or encourage sound sleep. Levels of light can also cause problems in the bedroom, including seemingly minor issues such as outdoor street lamps or alarm clock and cell phone lights. Window treatments and sleep masks can help to eliminate distracting light, allowing eyes, even when closed, to send messages to the brain that slumber is imminent. Noise levels should also be kept to a minimum, with the exception of white noise machines or other distractors, which can sometimes help to mask unwanted sounds.

> We found that all forms of noise in the sleep environment should be reduced to below 35 dB. The optimal ambient temperature varies based on humidity and the bedding microclimate, ranging between 17 and 28°C at 40–60% relative humidity. Complete darkness is optimal for sleep and blue light should be avoided during the sleep opportunity.
>
> (Caddick, Gregory, Arsintescu, & Flynn-Evans, 2018, p. 11)

Physical movement can be extremely beneficial for managing stress (see Chapter 3), but high intensity workouts completed too close to bedtime can disrupt sleep. When heart rate and blood pressure are increased, and body temperature spikes, it becomes both physically and mentally challenging to slow down enough to encourage sound sleep. Instead, aim for morning or early afternoon exercise, which will reap the full benefits of physical movement and actually encourage sleepiness at appropriate times of the evening. Stutz, Eiholzer, and Spengler (2018) performed a review of research literature regarding the impacts of evening exercise on sleep. Results of their review confirmed that exercise is indeed good for promoting onset of sleep, as well as quality of both REM and NREM rest throughout the night, but that vigorous exercise within an hour of bedtime can raise body temperature to the point of significant sleep disruption.

Exposure to natural light can also be a smart use of daytime physical movement. While sunscreen should be used, and sun exposure limited, daytime light (even on a cloudy day), will promote good physical and mental health. Duzgun and Durmaz (2017) examined the effects of sunlight on the sleep quality of "61 adults not diagnosed with major depression, not exercising regularly, not having sun allergy, not using sleeping pills, independent in activities of daily living, and having bad sleep quality" (p. 295). They exposed 30 experimental group participants to direct sunlight between the hours of 8:00 and 10:00 a.m. for five consecutive days, and found that the quality of nighttime sleep improved significantly compared to 31 control group participants.

In contrast to natural light, blue light from devices such as laptop computers, tablets, and smart phones can disrupt natural sleep processes by blocking melatonin release. Melatonin is a healthy chemical produced by the body to encourage normal sleep patterns. When it is masked by blue light, the brain receives messages to be more alert, even to the point of anxiety (National Sleep Foundation, 2019). Use of digital devices before bedtime can also disrupt sleep because of the nature of the content being consumed. Social media, email, and text messages can contain positive material, but more often include images and thoughts related to stress, manifested by an increase in physical and emotional tension (Walker, 2018). Despite these challenges, savvy use of technology can be beneficial for healthy sleep. Meditation apps such as "Calm" or "Headspace," white noise apps to block unwanted sound, display settings to limit the production of blue light, and even blogs or other online articles with sleep advice can aid in the quest for sound slumber (David, 2019).

Falling asleep can be difficult when attempted immediately following stressful work or anxious feelings. Therefore, it is important to slow down an hour or two before bedtime. Set a timer to intentionally stop checking email, social media, or anything work-related. Instead, try a warm shower or bath, do some light stretching and breathing exercises, or read a book for pleasure (being aware of potential light distractions if reading digitally). Similarly, once asleep, avoid the temptation to check clocks or phone notifications should you momentarily wake. It will be much easier to fall back asleep without these potential distractions. Finally, keep your sleeping space separate from other activities. Sound rest becomes difficult if the body has been sitting or lying in the same space while completing homework, watching television, or texting friends.

If it does become difficult to sleep after 20 minutes or more, calmly get out of bed and do something relaxing, like the activities mentioned in the preceding paragraph. Anxiously telling yourself to fall asleep will usually just make things worse, leading to even less sleep than becomes possible by getting up and returning soon after a calming activity. Very light snacks, such as a handful of healthy cereal or nuts, or a small glass of water or herbal tea, can also help to stave off hunger and lead more readily to slumber. Writing a short list of reminders or things to do can also help to relieve mental overload, allowing for more immediate sleep latency (National Sleep Foundation, 2019).

Mindfulness (see Chapter 7) can also be beneficial for healthy sleep. Ruminating thoughts before sleep or in the middle of the night can produce substantial challenges toward proper rest. When experiencing these thoughts, instead focus on parts of the body or patterns of breathing. Both can help to avoid judgmental focus on thoughts and associated worry about past or future events. Ong (2017) developed a treatment for chronic insomnia, mindfulness-based therapy for insomnia (MBTI). During the eight-week course, participants experience breathing and other meditation exercises, as well as cognitive strategies for identifying and managing thoughts that might disrupt sleep. As part of associated research studies, Ong found that MBTI actually increased brain activity in patients, suggesting that healthy sleep does indeed involve complex neural building and repair.

Breathe gently, focusing on the pattern of inhalation and exhalation. If thoughts enter your mind, simply observe them without judgment. You can even take some mild amusement from any mental block. Simply return to the pattern of inhalation and exhalation. Similarly, noticing different parts of the body, while keeping even breathing, can help to ease any unwanted physical tension. When performed with an easy sense of humor and a non-judging, non-striving attitude, these mindfulness activities will often help with drifting off to sleep (Migala, 2019).

In severe cases of insomnia, some people are tempted to try sleeping pills, and sometimes even receive prescriptions from medical professionals. However, these drugs should be considered as a last resort and, even then, treated with caution. "Sleeping pills do not provide natural sleep, can damage health, and increase the risk of life-threatening diseases" (Walker, 2018, p. 282). Walker went on to explain that, like alcohol, sleeping pills such as Ambien or Lunesta produce sedation, but not natural sleep. They will knock a person out, but the following hours will not allow the restorative REM and NREM functions of natural sleep, including memory consolidation, development of neural synapses, and emotional regulation. Sleeping pills are also often the cause of following day grogginess that can impair motor- and cognitive-skills. Huedo-Medina, Kirsch, Middlemass, Klonizakis, and Siriwardena (2012) conducted a review of research literature regarding the effectiveness of sleeping pills and found that placebos were statistically as effective as prescription medication for inducing sleep latency. "Scientific data on prescription sleeping pills suggests that they may not be the answer to returning sound sleep to those struggling to generate it on their own" (Walker, 2018, p. 284).

Revisiting the music education major, Zach, from the beginning of this chapter, let's consider how his life would be improved with better sleep. Zach still performs in a wind ensemble concert the night before his methods class, and helps to move percussion equipment afterwards. However, he has negotiated a rotation of responsibility with his studio professor and peers, such that he spends less time that night in exchange for other reasonable amounts of instrument maintenance throughout the semester. He politely declines the broomball invitation from his peers, telling them that he'll join them for basketball early the following afternoon. Because he has already eaten a healthy dinner before the concert, Zach returns to his dorm room, prepares a small cup of herbal tea, and takes a few minutes to review a summary of English exam notes, reassuring himself that previous study sessions have already prepared him well. Zach sends a couple of quick text messages to close friends and family, but resists the temptation to engross himself in social media, silencing phone notifications for the night. He closes the blinds, turns on a white noise machine, and takes a few minutes to breathe deeply. Zach is still a bit wound up after the exciting performance, so instead of being frustrated that he can't sleep, he turns on a soft light, reads a bit from a hard copy novel at his desk, and is soon feeling sleepy enough to nod off. Zach falls asleep around his regular time of 11:00–11:30 p.m. and wakes, without the aid of an alarm, at 7:00 a.m. He does some light stretching exercises, showers, walks to the dining hall for a good breakfast, and arrives ten minutes early at the music building, taking time to breathe and mentally prepare for what will prove to be a productive and engaging methods class.

Summary

- Aim for 7–9 hours of sleep per night.
- Keep a regular sleep schedule.
- Limit caffeine and alcohol.
- Avoid large meals close to bedtime.
- Exercise and seek natural light, but not too close to bedtime.
- Consider naps, but limit to around 30 minutes, not too close to bedtime.
- Keep the sleeping environment, cool, dark, and reserved for rest.
- Use a relaxing bedtime ritual, such as reading a book or meditating.

- If not asleep after 20–25 minutes, get out of bed, do something relaxing, and try again.
- Avoid digital distractions.
- Minimize prescription medications and report serious problems to a medical professional.

References

Barker, E. (2017). *Barking up the wrong tree: The surprising science behind why everything you know about success is (mostly) wrong.* New York, NY: Harper Collins.

Bentivoglio, M. & Grassi-Zucconi, G. (1997). The pioneering experimental studies on sleep deprivation. *Sleep, 20*(7), 570–576.

Buysse, D. J. (2014). Sleep health: Can we define it? Does it matter? *Sleep, 37*(1), 9–17.

Caddick, Z. A., Gregory, K., Arsintescu, L., & Flynn-Evans, E. E. (2018). A review of the environmental parameters necessary for an optimal sleep environment. *Building and Environment, 132*, 11–20.

Clark, I. & Landolt, H. P. (2017). Coffee, caffeine, and sleep: A systematic review of epidemiological studies and randomized controlled trials. *Sleep Medicine Reviews, 31*, 70–78.

David, N. (2019). 6 tech tips to get a better night's sleep. Retrieved September 1, 2019, from https://utswmed.org/medblog/6-tech-tips-get-better-nights-sleep/

Duzgun, G. & Durmaz, A. A. (2017). Effect of natural sunlight on sleep problems and sleep quality of the elderly staying in the nursing home. *Holistic Nursing Practice, 31*(5), 295–302.

Ebrahim, I. O., Shapiro, C. M., Williams, A. J., & Fenwick, P. B. (2013). Alcohol and sleep: Effects on normal sleep. *Alcoholism: Clinical and Experimental Research, 37*(4), 539–549.

Huedo-Medina, T. B., Kirsch, I., Middlemass, J., Klonizakis, M., & Siriwardena, A. N. (2012). Effectiveness of non-benzodiazepine hypnotics in treatment of adult insomnia: Meta-analysis of data submitted to the food and drug administration. *BMJ, 345*, e8343.

Jones, M. (2011, April 17). How little sleep can you get away with? *New York Times Magazine.*

Lightman, A. (2018). *In praise of wasting time.* New York, NY: Simon & Schuster.

Migala, J. (2019). 13 ways breathing better improves your life. In L. Lombardi (Ed.), *TIME special edition: The new mindfulness* (pp. 28–31). New York, NY: Meredith Corporation.

National Sleep Foundation. (2019). Retrieved August 18, 2019, from https://www.sleepfoundation.org/

Ong, J. C. (2017). *Mindfulness-based therapy for insomnia.* Washington, DC: American Psychological Association.

Pang, A. S. (2018). *Rest: Why you get more done when you work less.* New York, NY: Basic Books.

Patz, A. (2019). Sleep hacks for your most restful night ever. In L. Lombardi (Ed.), *TIME special edition: The new mindfulness* (pp. 86–91). New York, NY: Meredith Corporation.

Peterson, J. B. (2018). *12 rules for life: An antidote to chaos.* Toronto, ON: Random House Canada.

Rath, T. (2013). *Eat, move, sleep: How small choices lead to big changes.* San Jose, CA: Missionday.

Shojai, P. (2016). *The urban monk: Eastern wisdom and modern hacks to stop time and find success, happiness, and peace.* New York, NY: Rodale.

Stutz, J., Eiholzer, R., & Spengler, C. M. (2018). Effects of evening exercise on sleep in healthy participants: A systematic review and meta-analysis. *Sports Medicine, 49*(2), 269–287.

Wachob, J. (2016). *Wellth: How to build a life, not a résumé.* New York, NY: Harmony Books.

Wahlstrom, K. (2002). Changing times: Findings from the first longitudinal study of later high school start times. *NASSP Bulletin, 86*(633), 3–21.

Walker, M. (2018). *Why we sleep: Unlocking the power of sleep and dreams.* New York, NY: Scribner.

Walker, M. P. & Stickgold, R. (2010). Overnight alchemy: Sleep-dependent memory evolution. *Nature Reviews Neuroscience, 11*(218), 1–2.

Yoo, S., Gujar, N., Hu, P., Jolesz, F. A., & Walker, M. (2007). The human emotional brain without sleep: A prefrontal amygdala disconnect. *Current Biology, 17*(20), 877–878.

3 Physical Movement

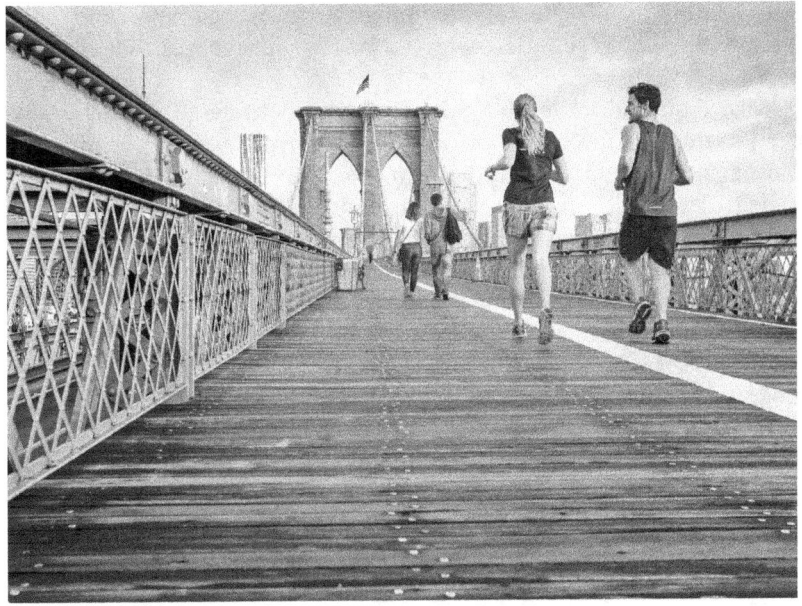

Figure 3.1 Physical movement
Source: Curtis Macnewton, Unsplash, https://unsplash.com/

Rhonda slumps in front of her piano, barely visible to her sixth period, middle school choir. She spends most of her teaching time on this piano bench, and otherwise sits at her desk, mindlessly completing administrative assignments, reviewing lesson plans, and sometimes finding time to surf the Internet. She doesn't even leave her classroom to eat lunch, instead opting to munch on processed snacks while completing other tasks. Rhonda notices dull pains creeping up her back, through her neck, and even behind her eyes, but simply pops a few Ibuprofen pills and keeps plugging along. Her general energy level is low, leading to apathetic classes and rehearsals. She barks some movement instructions to her students, related to an upcoming performance piece, but feels too sluggish to model the finished product. Friends of Rhonda have suggested that she join the local gym and complete a new fitness challenge that's trending on social media. But Rhonda simply rolls her eyes, insisting that she has never been athletic, can't afford a gym membership, and is far too tired to ever consider working out. Even when Rhonda does amble around her choir room, her movements are slow and laborious, mindlessly throwing herself around, breathing heavily, and stomping from foot to foot. By the middle of the school year, Rhonda's dull aches are becoming increasingly common and more intense. She has very little energy to muster, but realizes that changes are in order.

Like many music teachers, Rhonda has become so consumed by her job that she finds little or no time for formal exercise, or physical movement of any sort. While the term "exercise" is sometimes considered as negative or pejorative, physical movement is a very normal and essential part of the human condition (e.g., Rath, 2013; Wachob, 2016). In addition to maintaining and improving muscle function, heart health, and immune systems, moving ourselves improves brain processing and emotional health. "The neurons in the brain connect to one another through 'leaves' on treelike branches, and exercise causes those branches to grow and bloom with new buds, thus enhancing brain function at a fundamental level" (Ratey, 2008, p. 5). According to the United States Department of Health and Human Services (2019), over one-third of American adults are physically inactive and fewer than 5 percent exercise on a sustained basis, leading to severe problems with obesity, high blood pressure, high blood cholesterol, stroke, diabetes, heart disease, and cancer. "The average American commutes just under an hour per day and typically sits on a sofa watching 19.6 hours of TV per week … is it any wonder why we are gaining weight and stagnating?" (Shojai, 2016, p. 99). The Department of Health and Human Services recommends at least 30 minutes of physical movement every day, including aerobic, muscle-strengthening, bone-strengthening, balance, and stretching activities.

Physical movement can also help with sound sleep. According to the National Sleep Foundation (2019), a meta-analysis of research studies regarding the effects of exercise on sleep revealed increased total sleep time, improved NREM sleep, decreased REM sleep, and improved onset latency, the amount of time needed to fall asleep. However, caution should be applied to exercise too close to bedtime (less than three hours beforehand), as it will likely result in increased body temperature and disruption of sleep quality (Stutz, Eiholzer, & Spengler, 2018). Exercising outside can also be beneficial to sound sleep, as exposure to natural light promotes health (Duzgun & Durmaz, 2017). While exposure to natural light may be challenging during winter, it is still important to move as much as possible in this setting. On particularly cold days, it can help to start moving about inside in order to warm the body before heading outside.

Much recent work supports the positive impacts of physical movement on learning.

> When we exercise, particularly if the exercise requires complex motor movement, we're also exercising the areas of the brain involved in the full suite of cognitive functions. We're causing the brain to fire signals along the same network of cells, which solidifies their connections.
>
> (Ratey, 2008, p. 41)

Chang, Labban, Gapin, and Etnier (2012) conducted a review of 79 research studies regarding exercise and cognitive performance, and found positive effects during, immediately following, and after exercise. Etnier and Chang (2019) confirmed that the benefits of physical movement on cognition are evident for children, adolescents, adults, and seniors, and that there are benefits to be had from both short- and long-term fitness routines.

Physical movement helps to combat depression and anxiety. Anxiety is a natural response to stressful situations, intended to help the brain and body behave in appropriate ways to threats or other challenging situations. However, when this response occurs even without real threats, it can become uncomfortable and even debilitating. "Clinical anxiety affects about forty million Americans, or 18 percent of the population, in any given year and can manifest in a number of ways. They include generalized anxiety disorder, panic disorder, specific phobias, and social anxiety disorder" (Ratey, 2008, p. 87). State anxiety is a short-term response to threatening situations, while trait anxiety is a more constant feeling of stress regardless of context. Exercise helps with both situations, but, in particular, it eases false panic about a situation that is not actually threatening. By keeping cortisol in check and increasing the mood regulation of serotonin, regular physical movement balances emotional responses, allowing more accurate and calm assessments of perceived threats.

> "According to the World Health Organization, depression is the leading cause of disability in the United States and Canada, ahead of coronary heart disease, any given cancer, and AIDS. About 17 percent of American adults experience depression at some point in their lives.
>
> (Ratey, 2008, p. 114)

Regular physical movement encourages production of dopamine and endorphins, chemical reactions in the brain that dull pain and produce feelings of euphoria. Schuch, Vancampfort, Richards, Rosenbaum, Ward, and Stubs (2016) conducted a review of 25 research studies regarding the effects of exercise on depression. They found that aerobic exercise of moderate intensity was helpful in combating depression, particularly when supervised by professional trainers, and suggested that previous skeptical reports had been impacted by publication bias.

Similarly, physical movement can help to focus on the current moment.

> We frequently walk with the sole purpose of getting from one place to another. But where are we in between? With every step, we can feel the miracle of walking on solid ground. We can arrive in the present moment with every step.
>
> (Hanh, 2015, p. 8)

Too often, music teachers move through a school day without awareness, sitting stagnantly, moving mindlessly, worrying about what might be coming next, and simply trying to survive another day. However, by taking moments to focus on breathing and body awareness, mindful physical movements can help to relax and celebrate the gift of human embodiment.

> When you are alone, you can practice slow walking meditation. Choose a distance of about three meters, or ten feet, and as you traverse that distance, take one step for each in-breath and one step for each out-breath. With the first step you can say silently, "I have arrived." With the next step, you can say silently, "I am home." If you aren't arriving one hundred percent in the here and now, stay there and don't make another step. Challenge yourself. Breathe in and out again until you feel you have arrived one hundred percent in the here and the now. Then smile a smile of victory. Then make a second step. This is to learn a new habit, the habit of living in the present moment.
>
> (Hanh, 2015, p. 108)

As teaching careers progress, physical movement can help to curb stress and maintain appropriate health. "Exercise is one of the few ways to counter the process of aging because it slows down the natural decline of the stress threshold ... it increases blood volume, regulates fuel, and encourages neural activity and neurogenesis" (Ratey, 2008, pp. 223–224). Joseph, Adhihetty, and Leeuwenburgh (2017) found that both acute (short-term) and chronic (long-term) exercise can slow age-related deterioration of muscle health. Chou, Hwang, and Wu (2012) surveyed research conducted between 2001 and 2010 to determine the effects of exercise on physical function and the quality of life in older adults, and concluded that physical movement is beneficial to gait speed, coordination of balance, and performance in daily living activities.

Recommendations for Healthy Physical Movement

Before starting any program of physical movement, a medical professional should be consulted to ensure that the body is ready for routine exercise. Assuming that is the case, start slowly and make physical movement enjoyable. Part of the challenge with the term exercise is that many people assume it should be an awful form of drudgery. If you don't look forward to it, it's not likely to happen. Instead, choose activities that are enjoyable, such as chasing a frisbee, walking a dog, or playing catch. "Any amount of movement is better than none. And you can break it up into short bouts of activity throughout the day. Taking a brisk walk for five or ten minutes a few times a day will add up" (American Heart Association, 2019, p. 1). Lewis, Williams, Frayeh, and Marcus (2016) examined self-efficacy and perceived enjoyment as predictors of physical activity behavior and found perceived enjoyment to be the more important of the two. "Our results indicate that interventions should perhaps initially focus on increasing enjoyment of physical activity. Greater physical activity enjoyment appears to influence individuals' self-reported ability to engage in regular physical activity" (p. 456).

One method of increasing enjoyment of physical movement is by joining up with other people. "Seeking out like-minded people will help you make progress and keep you motivated and accountable to your physical activity program" (American Heart Association, 2019, p. 2). Local friends and family can be a particularly good place to start. Knowing that someone else is waiting on the corner outside your house serves as motivation to get out the door. Many area clubs, camps, and stores also offer opportunities for group yoga, running, moving meditation, and nature walking. Aral and Nicolaides (2017) examined exercise contagion among over one million runners across a five-year period and found that peer influence existed by ability level and gender. "Less active runners influence more active runners, while the reverse is not true. Both men and women influence men, while only women influence other women" (p. 1). Nielsen, Wikman, Jensen, Schmidt, Gliemann, and Andersen (2014) found that both enjoyment and social interaction were important factors in motivation to participate in physical movement. Participants in their study were more likely to continue physical activities when they involved extrinsic motivation of team sports (soccer), as opposed to needing intrinsic motivation of individual activities (spinning and crossfit).

Consulting a professional sports coach or personal trainer can also be beneficial to motivation, and can help to tailor specific activities related to age, fitness level, and personal goals. Dias, Simao, Saaverdra, and Ratamess (2017) studied the effects of a personal trainer on motivation and performance during strength training. Twenty-one participants completed leg presses, bench presses, leg extensions, and arm curls with and without the supervision of a personal trainer. Results indicated that personal trainers positively influenced self-selected training loads (motivation for level of weight) and ratings of perceived exertion. Local fitness centers often offer personal counseling and coaching services, or can provide references for other contacts.

Nutrition is important to consider during physical activities. Exercising when hungry can lead to lethargic efforts, and exercising when full, particularly with unhealthy foods, can lead to cramps and other physical feelings of distress. Maintaining proper levels of hydration is particularly important, especially in warm weather, but also at other times of the year. "A decrease in body water from normal levels (often referred to as dehydration or hypohydration) provokes changes in cardiovascular, thermoregulatory, metabolic, and central nervous function that become increasingly greater as dehydration worsens" (Murray, 2007, p. 5425). Furthermore, in a joint position paper of the American Dietetic Association, Dietitians of Canada, and American College of Sports Nutrition, Rodriguez, DiMarco, and Langley (2009) stated that "energy and macronutrient needs, especially carbohydrate and protein, must be met during times of high physical activity to maintain body weight, replenish glycogen stores, and provide adequate protein to build and repair tissue" (p. 709).

While many music teachers may prefer quiet environments when not at work, listening to music can have positive effects on exercise motivation and performance (e.g., American Heart Association, 2019). The psychological properties of pitch, rhythm, timbre, and loudness can interact for both sedative and stimulative effect, depending on the type of physical activity. Prabhakara and Farhan (2018) studied treadmill workouts of college students, and found that both maximum heart rate and exercise duration were better with music as opposed to no music. However, Nakamura, Pereira, Papini, Nakamura, and Kokubun (2010) found that unenjoyable music was worse than no music in the cycling efforts of adult participants. Music can be particularly useful for physical entrainment, matching exercise activities with particular tempi or beats per minute of music excerpts. Van Dyck, Moens, Buhmann, Demey, Coorevits, Dalla Bella, and Leman (2015) examined the effects of various music tempi on the gait of 16 recreational runners. They determined that changes in tempo of recorded music have a positive influence on running gait, which can help to modify steps and prevent or heal related injuries.

The American Heart Association (2019) recommended a blend of aerobic, strength, flexibility, and balance in physical movement. Examples of aerobic exercise include walking, running, swimming, and biking, and should be done for approximately 30 minutes per day, five days per week. Aerobic exercises temporarily increase breathing and heart rate to gradually improve the circulatory system. Strength and resistance exercises increase bone and muscle function, lowering the risk of injury, and improve metabolic rate, helping to burn calories more efficiently. "One set of eight to 12 repetitions, working the muscles to the point of fatigue, is usually sufficient for each muscle group" (American Heart Association, 2019, p. 5). Using a foam roller after aerobic and strength activities can aid in muscle recovery and physical comfort. Pearcey, Bradbury-Squires, Kawamoto, Drinkwater, Behm, and Button (2015) examined the effects of foam rolling as a recovery tool after intense exercise and found it to reduce delayed-onset muscle soreness 20 minutes, 24 hours, and 48 hours after exercise, compared to the absence of foam rolling. Similarly, Cheatham, Kolber, Cain, and Lee (2015) surveyed 14 research studies related to the benefits of foam rollers and roller massages and concluded that they can aid post-workout recovery and joint range of motion, but that they do not significantly improve performance when used before physical activity.

Balance and flexibility forms of physical movement are equally important, and can pair well with mindfulness activities (see aforementioned walking activities and Chapter 7). Balance activities can improve walking and stair climbing and can help to prevent unwanted falls. Yoga and tai chi are good formal balance exercises, but even walking in a straight line or standing on one foot for ten seconds can be beneficial. Similarly, remaining physically flexible is important for general health, and can be particularly important for musicians. Programs such as the Alexander Technique and the Feldenkrais Method involve specific exercises to improve flexibility and relieve pain or stress. "An Alexander

Technique teacher helps you to identify and lose the harmful habits you have built up over a lifetime of stress and learn to move more freely" (The Complete Guide to Alexander Technique, 2019, p. 1). Even short periods of light stretching can be beneficial for overall health.

> A stretch should always be smooth and slow, never jerky or bouncy. This can cause muscles to tighten and may result in injuries. Hold the stretch for 10–30 seconds and repeat each stretch 3–5 times. Remember to breathe normally during each stretch.
> (American Heart Association, 2019, p. 7)

Revisiting music teacher, Rhonda, from the beginning of this chapter, let's consider how her life would be improved with better physical movement. Rhonda still teaches her middle school choirs, but has replaced one piece per concert with an a cappella work, and has taught a few students from her keyboarding class to help with piano accompaniments. She is thus able to stand comfortably during the majority of rehearsals, mindfully conducting and modeling motions needed for some of the pieces. Between classes and rehearsals, Rhonda does a few light stretching and breathing exercises, and mindfully walks, at least three times per day, to the cafeteria, teachers' lounge, and main office. She builds a simple stand for her desk, such that she no longer needs to slump over computer keyboards or twist around tablets and smartphones. Rhonda challenges herself to park in remote parts of the school lot and completes some fun extracurricular walks with local friends and family. She has invested in a step-tracking watch, collecting at least 7,500 steps per day, and plans to join a local gym over the upcoming summer. Rhonda has just started a few low-intensity yoga classes, and is doing a bit of light weightlifting in the privacy of her own home. Most importantly, Rhonda is gaining confidence in the way she looks and feels, and is much happier in her job and life outside school.

Summary

- Consult a medical professional before starting any exercise routine.
- Make physical movement fun! If it's something you despise, you're less likely to do it.
- Keep a regular sleep schedule. Starting the day with some exercise can help to get going on a positive note.
- Get friends involved. Motivation from others can help to get out the door.
- Get outside as often as possible, even during the winter months.

- Exercise and seek natural light, but not too close to bedtime.
- Strive to do a mix of aerobic, strength, balance, and flexibility exercises.
- Use a foam roller or roller massager to aid muscle and joint recovery.
- Stay hydrated during physical activity, and choose foods that will power exercise.
- Practice mindful walking and be aware of breathing during physical movement.
- Find a coach. Informed professionals can design workouts geared to your needs.
- Embrace silence, but also consider music as a potential motivator for exercise.
- Count steps and embrace everyday activities as opportunities to move.

References

American Heart Association. (2019). Retrieved November 7, 2019, from https://www.heart.org/en/healthy-living/fitness/fitness-basics/aha-recs-for-physical-activity-in-adults

Aral, S., & Nicolaides, C. (2017). Exercise contagion in a global social network. *Nature Communications, 8,* 1–8.

Chang, Y. K., Labban, J. D., Gapin, J. I., & Etnier, J. L. (2012). The effects of acute exercise on cognitive performance: A meta-analysis. *Brain Research, 1453,* 87–101.

Cheatham, S. W., Kolber, M. J., Cain, M., & Lee, M. (2015). The effects of self-myofascial release using a foam roller or roller massager on joint range of motion, muscle recovery, and performance: A systematic review. *International Journal of Sports Physical Therapy, 10*(6), 827–838.

Chou, C. H., Hwang, C. L., & Wu, Y. T. (2012). Effect of exercise on physical function, daily living activities, and quality of life in the frail older adults: A meta-analysis. *Archives of Physical Medicine and Rehabilitation, 93*(2), 237–244.

The Complete Guide to the Alexander Technique. (2019). Retrieved November 12, 2019, from https://www.alexandertechnique.com

Dias, M. R., Simao, R. F., Saavedra, F. J., & Ratamess, N. A. (2017). Influence of a personal trainer on self-selected loading during resistance exercise. *The Journal of Strength and Conditioning Research, 31*(7), 1925–1930.

Duzgun, G. & Durmaz, A. A. (2017). Effect of natural sunlight on sleep problems and sleep quality of the elderly staying in the nursing home. *Holistic Nursing Practice, 31*(5), 295–302.

Etnier, J. L., & Chang, Y. K. (2019). Exercise, cognitive function, and the brain: Advancing our understanding of complex relationships. *Journal of Sport and Health Science, 8*(4), 299–300.

Hanh, T. N. (2015). *How to walk.* Berkeley, CA: Parallax Press.

Joseph, A. M., Adhihetty, P. J., & Leeuwenburgh, C. (2017). Beneficial effects of exercise on age-related mitochondrial dysfunction and oxidative stress in skeletal muscle. *The Journal of Physiology, 2*, 5105–5123.

Lewis, B. A., Williams, D. M., Frayeh, A., & Marcus, B. H. (2016). Self-efficacy versus perceived enjoyment as predictors of physical activity behavior. *Psychology & Health, 31* (4). 456–469.

Murray, B. (2007). Hydration and physical performance. *Journal of the American College of Nutrition, 26*, 5425–5485.

Nakamura, P. M., Pereira, G., Papini, C. B., Nakamura, F. Y., & Kokubun, E. (2010). Effects of preferred and nonpreferred music on continuous cycling exercise performance. *Perceptual and Motor Skills, 110*(1). 257–264.

National Sleep Foundation. (2019). Retrieved November 2, 2019, from https://www.sleepfoundation.org/articles/how-does-exercise-affect-sleep-duration-and-quality.

Nielsen, G., Wikman, J. M., Jensen, C. J., Schmidt, J. F., Gliemann, L., & Andersen, T. R. (2014). Health promotion: The impact of beliefs of health benefits, social relations and enjoyment on exercise continuation. *Scandinavian Journal of Medicine & Science in Sports, 24*(1), 66–75.

Pearcey, G. E., Bradbury-Squires, D. J., Kawamoto, J. E., Drinkwater, E. J., Behm, D. G., & Button, D. C. (2015). Foam rolling for delayed-onset muscle soreness and recovery of dynamic performance measures. *Journal of Athletic Training, 50*(1), 5–13.

Prabhakara, R. N., & Farhan, A. M. (2018). Effect of music on exercise performance in young adults. *International Journal of Physiology, 6*(4), 96–98.

Ratey, J. J. (2008). *Spark: The revolutionary new science of exercise and the brain.* New York, NY: Little, Brown Spark.

Rath, T. (2013). *Eat, move, sleep: How small choices lead to big changes.* San Jose, CA: Missionday.

Rodriguez, N. R., DiMarco, N. M., & Langley, S. (2009). American College of Sports Medicine position stand: Nutrition and athletic performance. *Medicine and Science in Sports and Exercise, 41*(3), 709–731.

Schuch, F. B., Vancampfort, D., Richards, J., Rosenbaum, S., Ward, P. B., & Stubs, B. (2016). Exercise as a treatment for depression. A meta-analysis adjusting for publication bias. *Journal of Psychiatric Research, 77*, 42–51.

Shojai, P. (2016). *The urban monk: Eastern wisdom and modern hacks to stop time and find success, happiness, and peace.* New York, NY: Rodale.

Stutz, J., Eiholzer, R., & Spengler, C. M. (2018). Effects of evening exercise on sleep in healthy participants: A systematic review and meta-analysis. *Sports Medicine, 49*(2), 269–287.

United States Department of Health and Human Services. (2019). Retrieved November 2, 2019, from https://www.hhs.gov/fitness/be-active/index.html

Van Dyck, E., Moens, B., Buhmann, J., Demey, M., Coorevits, E., Dalla Bella, S., & Leman, M. (2015). Spontaneous entrainment of running cadence to music tempo. *Sports Medicine Open, 1*(15), 1–14.

Wachob, J. (2016). *Wellth: How to build a life, not a résumé.* New York, NY: Harmony Books.

4 Nutrition

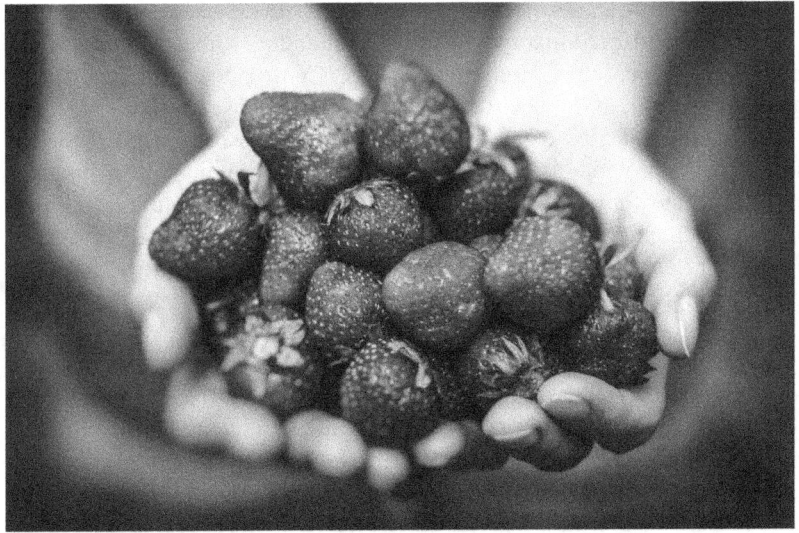

Figure 4.1 Nutrition
Source: Artur Rutkowski, Unsplash, https://unsplash.com/

Tony lies in his hospital bed, still unable to believe the doctors' news that his hip has been shattered. He had been rearranging marching band trophies the previous afternoon, when he felt a bit lightheaded and soon thereafter slipped off a stepladder, landing hard on the three-tiered floor of his rehearsal room. Tony is a dedicated high school band director, but has become somewhat obsessed with trophies and other awards, consistently demanding perfection from his students and himself. He always puts his job first, often at the expense of personal health and nutrition. While he is certainly not overweight, Tony struggles to consume sufficient macro and micronutrients, usually getting through a school day on nothing but coffee, soda, and an occasional sweet pastry. Evenings consist of mindlessly eating microwavable dinners, light beer, and snacks of salty chips and crackers, all consumed while answering emails and writing new drills for the next marching band season. The hospital doctors are surprised by the extent of hip damage from such a short fall, but after hearing details of Tony's diet, realize that he is severely dehydrated and lacking in major nutrients.

According to the Centers for Disease Control and Prevention, over one-third of American adults are obese, and from 1999–2000 to 2017–2018 the prevalence of obesity increased from 30.5 percent to 42.4 percent. "Obesity-related conditions include heart disease, stroke, type 2 diabetes and certain types of cancer that are some of the leading causes of preventable, premature death" (Centers for Disease Control and Prevention, 2020). Being underweight also poses health risks, and is often an indicator of poor nutrition. While visiting a professional health care provider is critical to address individual weight management, measuring body mass index (BMI) and waist circumference can be good starting points. The Centers for Disease Control and Prevention lists BMIs less than 18.5 as underweight, 18.5–24.9 as healthy, 25.0–29.9 as overweight, and 30.0 or above as obese.

> Fortunately, healthy nutrition can help to ameliorate obesity and other weight-related problems (e.g., Rath, 2013; Shojai, 2016; Wachob, 2016). Eating well can prevent 80 percent of heart attacks, 90 percent of type 2 diabetes, and 70 percent of colorectal cancer. It can also help you avoid stroke, osteoporosis, constipation and other digestive woes, cataracts, and age-related memory loss or dementia.
> (Willett & Skerrett, 2017, p. 1)

Many music educators struggle to find time for sound nutrition, and sometimes feel that they must fast or refrain from tasty food in order to be healthy. However, avoiding food will send messages to the brain that starvation is imminent, causing the body to hold on to fat and other calories. Limiting calories and trying faddy diets can also lead to psychological problems that will negatively affect other areas of health addressed in this book.

> A good diet should provide plenty of choices, relatively few restrictions, and no long lists of sometimes expensive special foods and supplements. It should be as good for your heart, bones, brain,

and colon as it is for your waistline. And it should be something you can sustain for years.

(Willett & Skerrett, 2017, p. 74)

One of the current challenges involves the proliferation of the processed food industry. From fast food chain restaurants to packaged foods in the aisles of traditional grocery stores, many dietary options are the antithesis of what human beings once consumed. Monteiro, Cannon, Levy, and Moubarac (2019) defined processed foods as those that are altered through chemical modification, fractioning of whole grains, and addition of artificial ingredients in an attempt to improve flavor, lower cost, and extend product shelf-life. They cautioned consumers to avoid unnatural food substances such as high-fructose corn syrup and chemical additives such as sweeteners, colors, and glazing agents.

Monteiro, Moubarac, Levy, and Canella (2018) found a clear link between household purchases of processed foods and rates of obesity, and recommended policy changes to encourage consumption of unprocessed foods and regulations to make processed foods less available and affordable. Similarly, Moubarac, Batal, Louzada, Steele, and Monteiro (2017) examined relationships between consumption of processed foods and dietary nutrient profiles, and found

> a significant and positive relationship between the dietary share of ultra-processed foods and the content in carbohydrates, free sugars, total and saturated fats and energy density, while an inverse relationship was observed with the dietary content in protein, fiber, vitamins A, C, D, B6 and B12, niacin, thiamine, riboflavin, as well as zinc, iron, magnesium, calcium, phosphorus and potassium.
>
> (p. 512)

Dehydration is another common challenge, caused by insufficient consumption of water and water-based foods. Stachenfeld, Leone, Mitchell, Freese, and Harkness (2018) conducted a study of 12 women related to daily intake of fluids and physical activity. They found that the participants did not consistently consume the recommended daily dose of fluid, and that they were, at times, dehydrated without being aware of the condition. Resultant challenges included decreases in visual and working memory, as well as executive function, but the researchers found that purposeful hydration improved both conditions. Regular hydration can also help to protect against the potential for future disease. For example, Carroll, Davis, and Papadaki (2015) found that plain water intake had a significant negative correlation with type 2 diabetes risk, and regression analysis suggested that water may have a direct role in that prevention.

A balanced diet consists of both macronutrients (carbohydrates, proteins, and fats) and micronutrients. "Vitamins and minerals are examples of micronutrients. While your body needs only small amounts of each vitamin and mineral, overall these micronutrients are vital to every bodily system and process" (Frazier, 2015, p. 11). Carbohydrates are a primary macronutrient for the body, and are typically referred to as simple or complex. Simple carbohydrates consist of just one or two sugar molecules, which allows for fast absorption, but can lead to unwanted peaks and valleys in energy. Examples include table sugar, refined white bread, and most snack chips and crackers. Complex carbohydrates consist of multiple sugar molecules, allowing for a more gradual and sustained release of energy throughout the day. Examples include whole grain oatmeal, brown rice, quinoa, and farro (Frazier, 2015). Shanahan and Shanahan (2016) and Willett and Skerrett (2017) cautioned that too many carbohydrates, primarily refined sugars, can increase the risk of obesity, as well as related health complications such as type 2 diabetes. "Sugar is the gateway drug. We now have research showing that exposure to sugar early in life has lasting effects on the brain that can make us more prone to developing chemical dependencies" (Shanahan & Shanahan, 2016, p. 222).

"Proteins are composed of long chains of amino acids and are present in every cell in the body … the body uses protein quickly, requiring a consistent supply from food sources" (Frazier, 2015, p. 53). Willett and Skerrett (2017) recommended consuming protein from plant sources such as beans and nuts, or from lean animal sources such as fish or chicken. Dairy can also be a good source of protein, and calcium, but recent recommendations from health experts have suggested that too much could have harmful effects.

> Dairy is in a class by itself, with about 300 milligrams of calcium per glass of milk or the equivalent amount of cheese or yogurt. Adding one serving of milk, yogurt, or other dairy food a day will almost certainly ensure you get the calcium you need.
> (Willett & Skerrett, 2017, p. 204)

Fats are essential for healthy nutrition. While sometimes blamed for weight gain and other challenges, monounsaturated fats such as fresh salmon, olive oil, avocados, and almonds contain important nutrients that are crucial for a healthy body (Frazier, 2015). In fact, low-fat diets often deplete humans of these critical nutrients, replacing them with dangerous sugars, partially hydrogenated vegetable oils, and other chemicals. Artificial trans fats are indeed a poor source of calories. "These include margarines, vegetable shortenings, doughnuts, commercial baked goods such as packaged pastries and cookies, powdered creamer, and the fats used for deep-frying fast food in restaurants" (Willett & Skerrett, 2017, p. 83). But while trans fats are certainly to be avoided, monounsaturated fats are an important component of balanced health.

Recommendations for Healthy Nutrition

Visiting a primary doctor or nutrition specialist should be a basic starting point for assessing current dietary needs. Variables related to current health and family history can influence individual requirements. However, general best practices have been outlined by the United States Department of Agriculture (2020). In addition to approximately 64 ounces of water per day, they recommend a "my plate plan" balancing fruits, vegetables, grains, protein, and dairy. A customizable version of their plan is available at choosemyplate.gov, offering specific recommendations based on age, gender, and typical physical activity. Tips regarding meal preparation, snack options, shopping for local ingredients, and connections to exercise are also available on the website.

While in agreement with most of these guidelines, Willett and Skerrett (2017) suggested less emphasis on carbohydrates, particularly those that are processed and refined, and more consumption of healthy fats, such as nuts, avocadoes, salmon, and olive oil, as well as lean sources of protein, such as fish and poultry. They provided the following guidelines:

> Celebrate vegetables and fruits: Cover half of your plate with them. Aim for color and variety. Keep in mind that potatoes don't count.
>
> Go for whole grains – about one-quarter of your plate. Intact and whole grains, such as whole wheat, barley, wheat berries, quinoa, oats, brown rice, and foods made with them, have a milder effect on blood sugar and insulin than white bread, white rice, and other refined grains.
>
> Choose healthy protein packages – about one-quarter of your plate. Fish, chicken, beans, soybeans, and nuts are all healthy, versatile protein sources. Limit red meat, and try to stay away from processed meats such as bacon and sausage.
>
> Use healthy plant oils, such as olive, canola, soy, corn, sunflower, and peanut, in moderation. Stay away from foods containing partially hydrogenated oils, which contain unhealthy artificial trans fats. If you like the taste of butter or coconut oil, use them when

their flavor is important but not as primary dietary fats. Keep in mind that low-fat does not mean healthy.

Drink water, coffee, or tea. Skip sugary drinks. If you enjoy milk, don't have more than two glasses a day. If you drink alcohol, keep it moderate – no more than two drinks a day for men, no more than one a day for women.

Exercise. It's good for overall health and controlling weight.

(pp. 4–5)

Eating early in the day can be particularly important in the teaching profession. Waking up at the last minute, rushing to school, and attempting to teach on an empty stomach will often lead to lack of energy, and will promote binge eating later in the day. Similarly, eating and drinking late in the evening will make it difficult to fall asleep and will disrupt quality of sleep throughout the night. Kaczmarek, Musaad, and Holscher (2017) found that eating early positively affected the composition and function of gut microbes, while Walker, Christopher, Wieth, and Buchanan (2015) found that "morningness" predicted healthy eating patterns and "eveningness" predicted neuroticism and unhealthy eating patterns. Mindfully consuming a balanced breakfast of whole, complex carbohydrates with some protein and healthy fat ensures a slow release of energy throughout the day. For example, whole grain oatmeal with some raisins and soy protein, or whole grain crackers with natural peanut butter and a side of fruit and yogurt, are both relatively easy meals to prepare and digest before heading out the door.

Once at school, it can be useful to consume healthy snacks and water throughout the day. Nicklas, O'Neil, and Fulgoni (2014) examined the impacts of snacking patterns on the health of 18,988 adults. The researchers suggested that snacking is better than no snacking, but that choices of vegetables, legumes, whole fruit, and milk had better impacts on health than the more popular choices of cakes, cookies, pastries, and sodas. While visiting the school cafeteria or faculty room can be socially healthy, avoid temptations to consume processed foods just because they are available. Birthday cakes and doughnuts, high-sodium cafeteria meals, and unhealthy vending machine options are typical staples of school environments, but will ultimately lead to waves of sugar highs and energy lows. Instead, pack small containers of balanced snacks and lunch. Nuts, whole grains such as brown rice or quinoa, fresh fruit, and sliced vegetables can all be easily consumed in short breaks between classes. Keeping a reusable water bottle nearby gives opportunities to sip slowly, remain hydrated, and encourage vocal health.

Monitoring serving sizes is also important. Be mindful of nutrition labels to be sure that a bowl of cereal or dinner preparation of pasta does not contain multiple servings. Rosenthal and Raynor (2017) found that adult participants were much more likely to consume extra calories when presented with large versus small servings of food. Restaurant portions are notoriously large, particularly for dinner servings. Asking for half of a meal to be packaged for later consumption can help avoid the temptation to inadvertently consume too many servings.

Eating mindfully, both at school and at home, can provide space for enjoyment of various aromas, textures, and flavors, as well as allowing space for healthy digestion. "Mindful eating generally refers to the application of mindfulness techniques to eating, which involves non-judgmental awareness of internal and external cues influencing the desire to eat, food choice, quantity of consumption, and the manner in which food is consumed" (Fung, Long, Hung, & Cheung, 2016). Rogers and Maytan (2012) recommended the following meditation, using a single grape or raisin, to encourage mindful eating.

> Please get into your meditation position with your eyes closed. Let your hands rest quietly in your lap, one hand on top of the other, palms up. I am going to place an object in your hand, and I want you to let it rest there without any movement. Now, bring your awareness to the object. What does it feel like? What is the texture, the temperature, the weight? Do you notice your mind wondering what it might be or thinking that you know what it is? Now, open your eyes and bring your full attention to the object resting in your hand. Notice the color. Notice if the light shines on it differently in different places. Notice if there are smooth or rough places. Pretend that you have just landed on this planet and you have never seen an object like this. Notice any thoughts you are having as you look at the object. Are there any sensations in your mouth that might be signaling a wish to eat the object? Are you wondering what the point of this is? Are you waiting for this exercise to be over? Just notice the thoughts and bring your attention to the object. Now, I'm about to tell you to bring the object up under your nose. Remember to concentrate on every movement it takes to move your hand and arm. Okay, go ahead. Just hold the object under your nose and notice the smell, what is happening in your mouth, your thoughts …. Then slowly open your mouth and place the object in it without chewing or swallowing it. Just let it rest in your mouth and notice everything that is happening in your mouth. Do you notice a desire to chew? Do you notice impatience? Do you notice salivation? Now, begin to chew very slowly and mindfully, noticing the taste, your

tongue movements, texture, changes in texture and taste. Do not swallow yet .... Finally, you may begin to swallow. See if you feel the bits of food as they go down your esophagus.

(pp. 115–116)

Limit or avoid caffeine and alcohol, as both dehydrate the body and cause disruption to normal energy levels. While caffeine can feel like a pleasant, and perhaps necessary, part of a music teacher's morning routine, too much of the stimulant can cause an unnatural spike in adrenaline, followed by a sudden feeling of sleepiness. Caffeine too late in the day can also cause disruptions to normal sleeping patterns. "In a nutshell, it can be said that caffeine acts as a boon as well as bane because it possesses both beneficial and adverse effects" (Kumar, Kaur, Panghal, Kaur, & Handa, 2018). Similarly, alcohol will disrupt sleep, particularly when consumed in large quantities. While it may be tempting to enjoy a glass of wine or beer after a stressful day of teaching, and it may feel as though the alcohol is making you sleepy, disruption of slumber will occur when the alcohol wears off, usually at some point in the middle of the night. Thus, what might look like a solid seven or eight hours of sleep will feel more like five or six.

Shop the perimeters of grocery stores to seek a colorful variety of natural, sustainably produced nutrition. While exceptions to the rule exist, most traditional supermarkets include natural foods such as fruit, vegetables, meats, and dairy around the outer walls of the building. More processed foods, containing additives intended to increase shelf life, are usually housed in the aisles of the store. "Many Western diseases such as heart disease, stroke, cancer, diabetes, and arthritis are a result of the additives in our food and preservatives used" (Benson, 2019, p. 20). Similarly, seek foods that contain very short lists of ingredients, and pay particular attention to the first ingredients listed. Whole grains or fruits without extra ingredients are much better for human health than products with long lists of terms such as refined white flour, added sugars, and processed vegetable oils. Benson (2019) supported these notions, stating that "a key piece of advice is to make your diet simple, just shop the perimeters of the supermarket and avoid the packaged foods in the aisles of the store" (p. 20).

Despite the aforementioned recommendations, it is indeed okay, and even psychologically beneficial, to enjoy an occasional treat. Savoring a small piece of chocolate, a cup of coffee or glass of wine, or even a less healthy snack, appetizer, or dessert on occasion can provide a welcome break from clean eating, and can sometimes even introduce healthy levels of dietary variety. Considering other areas of health introduced in this book, "cheat meals" or other treats can also offer extended opportunities for gratitude, pleasure, and mindfulness. However, consuming treats in small quantities can sometimes lead down a path of binge eating and drinking. Consider enjoying treats only outside of home and work environments. If such temptations are readily available in a house or school building, they are much more likely to be consumed on a regular basis. You may curse the lack of available treats during moments of weakness, but will ultimately be grateful to have been guided into a healthier choice.

Revisiting high school band director, Tony, let's consider how his personal and professional experiences might be improved through better nutrition. Tony admires the few marching band trophies that are displayed around his band room, but feels healthy and fulfilled enough to realize that there is more to the program than awards and accolades. As students enter the band room for morning rehearsal, Tony slowly sips on the last bit of a fruit and protein smoothie he had prepared before school. At lunchtime, he enjoys a relaxed conversation with colleagues as he mindfully consumes a quinoa and salmon salad. After munching on a light snack of almonds and raisins during afternoon marching band rehearsal, making sure to also drink plenty of water, Tony enjoys a balanced dinner of chicken, broccoli, and farro, leaving sufficient time for digestion before heading to bed. While still respected and admired by his students and other members of the local community, Tony appreciates his newfound levels of energy, feeling calm and in control of his life, both personal and professional.

Summary

- Enjoy a balanced diet of real food. It should taste good!
- Eat early in the day. Eating and drinking late at night can disrupt sleep.
- Eat slowly and mindfully. Enjoy the process.
- Consume several small meals and nutritious snacks throughout the day.
- Monitor serving sizes. Restaurant and self-created portions are often too large.
- Hydrate with water on a regular basis. Limit or avoid caffeine and alcohol.
- Shop on the perimeters of grocery stores. Seek natural foods.
- Enjoy whole and colorful foods from sustainable sources.
- Balance the macronutrients of carbohydrates, proteins, and fats.
- Balance the micronutrients of vitamins and minerals by consuming a variety of foods.
- Enjoy treats in moderation.

References

Benson, D. (2019). Eat like a caveman. *Alternative Medicine, 46,* 20–21.

Carroll, H. A., Davis, M. G., & Papadaki, A. (2015). Higher plain water intake is associated with lower type 2 diabetes risk: A cross-sectional study in humans. *Nutritional Research, 35*(10), 865–872.

Centers for Disease Control and Prevention. (2020). Retrieved March 5, 2020, from https://www.cdc.gov/obesity/index.html

Frazier, K. (2015). *Nutrition facts: The truth about food.* Berkeley, CA: Rockridge Press.

Fung, T. T., Long, M. W., Hung, P., & Cheung, L. W. Y. (2016). An expanded model for mindful eating for health promotion and sustainability: Issues and challenges for dietetics practice. *Journal of the Academy of Nutrition and Dietetics, 116*(7), 1081–1086.

Kaczmarek, J. L., Musaad, S. M. A., & Holscher, H. D. (2017). Time of day and eating behaviors are associated with the composition and function of the human gastrointestinal microbiota. *The American Journal of Clinical Nutrition, 106*(5), 1220–1231.

Kumar, V., Kaur, J., Panghal, A., Kaur, S., & Handa, V. (2018). Caffeine: A boon or bane. *Nutrition and Food Science, 48*(1), 61–75.

Monteiro, C. A., Cannon, G., Levy, R. B., & Moubarac, J. C. (2019). Ultra-processed foods: What they are and how to identify them. *Public Health Nutrition, 22*(5), 936–941.

Monteiro, C. A., Moubarac, J. C., Levy, R. B., & Canella, D. S. (2018). Household availability of ultra-processed foods and obesity in nineteen European countries. *Public Health Nutrition, 21*(1), 18–26.

Moubarac, J. C., Batal, M., Louzada, M. L., Steele, E. M., & Monteiro, C. A. (2017). Consumption of ultra-processed foods predicts diet quality in Canada. *Appetite, 108*(1), 512–520.

Murray, B. (2007). Hydration and physical performance. *Journal of the American College of Nutrition, 26,* 542S–548S.

Nicklas, T. A., O'Neil, C. E., & Fulgoni, V. L. (2014). Snacking patterns, diet quality, and cardiovascular risk factors in adults. *BMC Public Health, 14,* 388.

Rath, T. (2013). *Eat, move, sleep: How small choices lead to big changes.* San Jose, CA: Missionday.

Rogers, H. B., & Maytan, M. (2012). *Mindfulness for the next generation: Helping emerging adults manage stress and lead healthier lives.* New York, NY: Oxford University Press.

Rosenthal, R. & Raynor, H. (2017). The effect of television watching and portion size on intake during a meal. *Appetite, 117*(1), 191–196.

Shanahan, C. & Shanahan, L. (2016). *Deep nutrition: Why your genes need traditional food.* New York, NY: Flatiron Books.

Shojai, P. (2016). *The urban monk: Eastern wisdom and modern hacks to stop time and find success, happiness, and peace.* New York, NY: Rodale.

Stachenfeld, N. S., Leone, C. A., Mitchell, E. S., Freese, E., & Harkness, L. (2018). Water intake reverses dehydration associated impaired executive function in healthy young women. *Physiology & Behavior, 185*(1), 103–111.

United States Department of Agriculture. (2020). Retrieved March 19, 2020, from https://www.choosemyplate.gov/resources/MyPlatePlan

Wachob, J. (2016). *Wellth: How to build a life, not a résumé.* New York, NY: Harmony Books.

Walker, R. J., Christopher, A. N., Wieth, M. B., & Buchanan, J. (2015). Personality, time-of-day preference, and eating behavior: The mediational role of morning-eveningness. *Personality and Individual Differences, 77,* 13–17.

Willett, W. & Skerrett, P. (2017). *Eat, drink and be healthy: The Harvard Medical School guide to healthy eating.* New York, NY: Simon & Schuster.

5 Gratitude

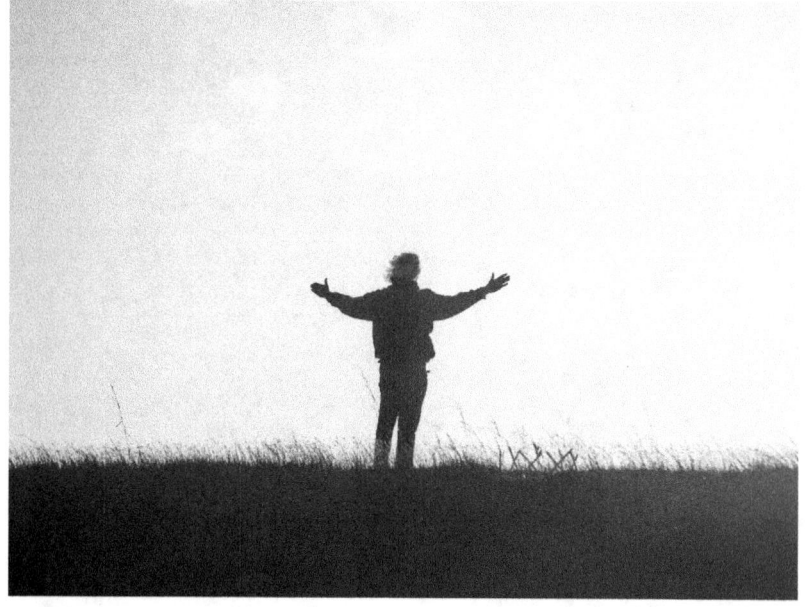

Figure 5.1 Gratitude
Source: Debby Hudson, Unsplash, https://unsplash.com/

Paul angrily slams his phone down, frustrated that no one has liked or commented on his latest Facebook post. He looks around his university office, wondering whether he made a mistake in pursuing a doctoral degree and moving into higher education. A mountain of papers waits to be graded, syllabi for the next semester need to be prepared, and Paul frets that his recent research manuscript submission will be rejected. He longs for his days of teaching high school and middle school orchestra, remembering only the best moments from that decade of his career. From an outside perspective, Paul seems to have a great situation, having recently been hired to a tenure track assistant professor position in string education at a thriving School of Music in a charming small town. His university students are inquisitive, musical, and hardworking, and they all seem to enjoy working with Paul, praising his sense of humor, playing abilities, and academic knowledge. However, instead of focusing on the positive, Paul can only perceive the challenging parts of his life, longing for life in a big city, wishing he had more friends, scanning digital news feeds for negative stories, and anxiously worrying about the future. Instead of expressing thanks for everything he has, Paul retreats into solitude most days and nights, venting on social media, and feeling rather hopeless.

Like many others, Paul fails to notice the good in life, missing positive moments while focusing on the negative.

> When we neglect gratitude, we are, in effect making a choice toward negative emotions, which in turn foster more negativity. But when, if even for a little while, we choose gratefulness, that choice builds on itself and begins to create a spiral of appreciation.
>
> (Bass, 2018, p. 88)

Experts from the field of positive psychology have suggested that practicing gratitude, or a feeling of thanksgiving, can help teachers manage stress and prevent burnout (e.g., Emmons, 2007; Seligman, 2011). McCullough, Emmons, and Tsang (2002) found gratitude to be positively related to optimism and life satisfaction, while negatively related to depression, anxiety, materialism, and envy. Emmons (2007) further documented that gratitude can enhance willpower, improve creativity, deepen spirituality, increase self-esteem, and even enhance academic performance. Algoe, Haidt, and Gable (2008) examined the effects of gift-giving and found that generosity and gratitude were both helpful with the formation and maintenance of positive personal relationships. "The ability to feel grateful is a huge part of enjoying satisfaction in life. If we can't feel gratitude, we're locking ourselves out of one of the most important and uplifting aspects of well-being" (Wachob, 2016, p. 179).

Bass (2018) noted that traditional notions of gratitude often involve benefactors and beneficiaries, in a targeted, controlled system of giving with expectation for reciprocity. In worst-case scenarios, she continued, those on the receiving end are indebted to their givers, potentially leading to guilt and shame. But when gifts are recognized as naturally occurring in the existing world, the practice of gratitude can shift to untargeted recognition, appreciation, and positive response. "In this mode, gifts exist before benefactors. The universe is a gift. Life is a gift. Air, light, soil, and water are gifts … Everything we need is here, with us" (Bass, 2018, p. xxiv).

In a four-tier model, Bass suggested that gratitude includes personal and communal expressions, with both emotional feeling and ethical response. Personal emotions of gratitude might include strong feelings of awe, delight, and joy when someone helps or offers a gift of some sort. Ethical response from a personal perspective involves traditional reciprocation, often in the form of a spoken "thanks" or a more formal email, text message, or hand-written card. Communal, emotional expressions of gratitude often occur in places of worship or at sporting events, as large groups gather to express common thanks through prayer, music, or cheer. Finally, expressions of gratitude through communal ethics result in civic commitments to volunteerism, charity, and stewardship (Bass, 2018).

Bass cautioned that gratitude should not be oversimplified, and can be difficult to negotiate in cases of deep sickness or trauma. Suffering individuals will likely need physical and/or mental therapy to address underlying tensions before normal practices of gratitude can be appreciated. She also noted that males often struggle with gratitude more than females. Kashdan, Mishra, Breen, and Froh (2009) supported this notion in a series of studies related to gender and gratitude. They found that women, compared with men, found gratitude more rewarding and expressed it more easily. Men reported greater feelings of burden and obligation than women after receiving a gift. "Women with greater gratitude were more likely to satisfy needs to belong and feel autonomous; gratitude had the opposite effect in men" (p. 691).

Despite these cautions, gratitude has been found to be beneficial across various populations. For example, Froh, Sefick, and Emmons (2008) examined the effects of gratitude on the subjective well-being of 221 early adolescents. They assigned participants randomly to one of three groups (gratitude, hassles, or control), and found that counting one's blessings improved school experience immediately following treatment and the three weeks following. Toepfer, Cichy, and Peters (2012) studied the effects of writing letters of gratitude. Middle-aged adult participants wrote three letters over a period of three weeks and reported increased happiness and life-satisfaction, as well as decreased depression. Similarly, Killen and Macaskill (2015) found two weeks of gratitude journaling to be beneficial for older adults, both short-term and one month following treatment.

Olympic athlete Deena Kastor found that gratitude helped push her beyond pure physical prowess and running talent. She knew that physical training alone was not enough to succeed at an international level, and she was feeling burned out in the process. But adding readings and mental practices related to positivity and gratitude helped Kastor to remember childlike pleasures in running, enabling her to notice enjoyment and thrive in competitions. "Constantly scanning the world for goodness, I ran with greater lightness, infused with a deep appreciation for Coach, everyone around me, the opportunities before me, and my body itself. Positive thoughts came more quickly now, without a conscious shift" (Kastor & Hamilton, 2018, p. 97).

The Gratitude Questionnaire – Six Item Form is a survey developed by McCullough, Emmons, and Tsang (2002) that has been employed in research studies to measure gratefulness among various populations (Table 5.1). I used the survey in two recent studies of music majors and K-12 music educators. Participants for the first study (Bernhard, 2020) were 257 music majors at a public university school of music (47.07 percent of 546 potential respondents) who were compared by year in school (freshman, sophomore, junior, senior, or graduate) and major (music education or non-music education). The secondary purpose was to examine the relationship between perceived gratitude and academic/personal variables (number of credits and hours per week of classes, ensembles, homework, practice, exercise, sleep, work, and socializing). Collectively, mean scores for gratitude were comparable to university students in previous studies (e.g., Kashdan, Mishra, Breen, & Froh 2009; McCullough, Emmons, & Tsang, 2002). The results of

Table 5.1 The Gratitude Questionnaire – Six Item Form (GQ–6)

1 = strongly disagree 2 = disagree 3 = slightly disagree 4 = neutral 5 = slightly agree 6 = agree 7 = strongly agree

1. I have so much in life to be thankful for.
2. If I had to list everything that I felt grateful for, it would be a very long list.
3. When I look at the world, I don't see much to be grateful for.*
4. I am grateful to a wide variety of people.
5. As I get older I find myself more able to appreciate the people, events, and situations that have been part of my life history.
6. Long periods of time can go by before I feel grateful for something or someone.*

Scoring Instructions:
1. Add your scores for items 1, 2, 4, and 5.
2. Reverse your scores for items 3 and 6. That is, if you scored a "7," give yourself a "1," if you scored a "6," give yourself a "2," etc.
3. Add the reversed scores for items 3 and 6 (marked with asterisk) to the total from Step 1. This is your total GQ–6 score. This number should be between 6 and 42.

Source: McCullough, Emmons, and Tsang (2002, p. 87)

multivariate and univariate analyses of variance revealed that no significant differences in gratitude were reported by year in school, but music education majors reported significantly higher levels of gratitude than non-music education majors. Moderate positive correlations were observed between gratitude and reported hours of sleep. It's no surprise that those who reported more sleep were also likely to report stronger dispositions for gratitude, and it's promising for the teaching profession that music education majors were more likely than other music majors to feel grateful.

Participants for the second study (Bernhard, 2019) were 235 music teachers from the state of New York (47 percent of 500 potential respondents) who were compared by grade level taught (elementary, middle, high school, or a combination), certification status (initial or professional), and teaching area (instrumental, choral/general, or a combination). The secondary purpose was to examine the relationship between perceived gratitude and teaching/personal variables (number of hours per week of teaching, preparing, exercising, sleeping, socializing, family obligations, and doing another job). Collectively, mean scores for gratitude were comparable to adults in previous studies (e.g., Giacalone, Paul, & Jurkiewicz, 2005; McCullough, Emmons, & Tsang, 2002). Results of multivariate and univariate analyses of variance revealed that middle school music teachers reported lower levels of gratitude than other music educators, and early career music teachers (four or fewer years in the profession) reported lower levels of gratitude than those with more experience. Regarding teaching area, instrumental music teachers reported higher levels of gratitude than others, on average. Moderate positive correlations were observed between gratitude and reported hours of exercise, while moderate negative correlations were observed between gratitude and hours of teaching preparation. Support for early career teachers, as well as those who teach middle grades and/or a combination of general/choral is likely needed, as is further education about the importance of exercise and work-life balance.

Recommendations for Practicing Gratitude

One of the first steps in practicing gratitude is developing awareness. Recommendations from the mindfulness chapter of this book could be a good start, leading to what professionals refer to as "gratitude interventions" (Bass, 2018, p. 55). To further assist in developing awareness of positive events and circumstances, setting specific times and practices can be helpful. For example, starting or ending each day by identifying one source of gratitude can be beneficial. "Not only is this a beneficial spiritual practice; several scientific studies have shown that people who practice gratitude right before bedtime sleep better, more soundly, and more deeply" (Bass, 2018, p. 80). Some find it useful to say or sing a grace before meals. Others focus on gratitude while walking or meditating. In a series of eight research studies, Lambert, Fincham, and Stillman (2012) found that interventions such as gratitude journaling are related to reduction in depressive symptoms by way of reframing negative thoughts and promoting positive emotions. The act of writing, particularly on hard copy, allows time for thought and reflection, delving more deeply into reasons for thanks in comparison to simply thinking about gratitude. "Include at least three items ... it takes three to five positive thoughts or feelings to counter negativity. Avoid repeating the same items because it challenges you to look for gratitude in unexpected or surprising places" (Kastor & Hamilton, 2018, p. 87).

Gratitude practices can offer opportunities for contemplation of the past, present, and future. Gratitude for the past includes recognition of privilege and love received from others, such as parents, siblings, or lifelong friends. Care should be exercised to avoid dramatizing past events through rose-colored glasses. Nostalgic recall of only positive events can lead to distress and longing for the past. Instead, balance realistic reflection, noting the opportunities for thanksgiving. Future planning can also be a place for gratitude, recognizing any potential opportunity for success and happiness. As with reflection about past events, care should be taken to avoid anxiously spinning out of control regarding events and other circumstances that have yet to materialize. Most importantly, gratitude for the current moment can offer an opportunity for stress release and focus. Calm awareness of the present moment leads to savoring of the good. Focus on what currently is and how it might be better than other alternatives. "Yes, gratitude still holds the power to surprise and to elicit a strong emotional response. However, as a habit, it also becomes a steadying companion, incorporated into the story of our lives" (Bass, 2018, p. 86).

Similarly, researchers and other scholars have discussed the notion of tailwinds versus headwinds. While it is sometimes easier to notice headwinds, or life's difficulties and challenges, recognizing tailwinds, opportunities and advantages that are already in place, can be equally or more beneficial. Davidai and Gilovich (2016) conducted seven research studies to investigate how headwind (barrier) and tailwind (blessing) perceptions might operate in daily life. Among their findings, they stated that "Democrats and Republicans both claim that the electoral map works against them ... and academics think that they have a harder time with journal reviewers, grant panels, and tenure committees than members of other subdisciplines" (p. 835). Similarities might occur for music educators, who often perceive that they are underfunded, unnoticed, and underappreciated. At the same time, they may fail to recognize that other teachers are often jealous that the arts are not required to undergo standardized testing and that there is a perceived benefit in having curricular flexibility. Davidai and Gilovich suggested that by purposely focusing on tailwind blessings, it might be possible to identify and manage headwind bias.

Bono (2020) presented a similar concept when writing about gratitude in relation to happiness and positive psychology. He suggested that life satisfaction can be measured as a mathematical equation of division, in which recognizing what we have serves as the numerator, and pining for what we think we want serves as the denominator. For example, five blessings that are already occurring versus one item of want would result in a life satisfaction, or happiness, score of five. Recognizing only one blessing while longing for five items of want would result in a happiness score of only 0.20, or one-fifth of one. "Our happiness depends not only on what our lives are *actually* like, but also what we *want* them to be like" (p. 30). "It shouldn't shock us that as our sense of entitlement increases, our happiness decreases. In fact, disappointment replaces happiness because we feel we are constantly failing to receive benefits we should be receiving" (Elmore & McPeak, 2019, p. 121).

Another method for enhancing the practice of thanksgiving is by joining other people. "Gratitude takes us outside ourselves, where we see ourselves as part of a larger, intricate network of sustaining relationships, relationships that are mutually reciprocal" (Emmons, 2007, p. 54). Environments such as sporting events, political rallies, and music concerts can provide rich opportunities for communal thanksgiving. However, Bass (2018) cautioned that situations in which some win while others lose often lead to feelings of disappointment, jealousy, and resentment, the antitheses of gratitude. Given this consideration, perhaps it is important for music teachers to carefully examine the role of competition in classroom and rehearsal settings. Seating auditions, solo and ensemble festivals, and major concerts can all be wonderful learning opportunities, and are certainly authentic to the profession. But when allowed to fester out of control, they can lead to undue distress and anxiety for students and teachers alike.

> If you are thankful for something that cuts you off from others or sets people at odds, it may not be genuine gratitude. It may be an emotion birthed in fear and control. Gratitude connects us, even across racial, class, and national boundaries, allowing us to *feel* together.
>
> (Bass, 2018, p. 107)

In addition to the potential negative aspects of competition, loneliness is a challenge that faces an increasing number of individuals. As a result of sprawling suburbs and the impact of technology, more and more people are feeling isolated and alone (Bass, 2018). Caputo (2015) affirmed this situation, but suggested that gratitude could be beneficial. In a web-based survey of 197 participants, she found a negative correlation between gratitude and loneliness, and suggested that "gratitude succeeds in accounting for up to almost one-fifth of the total variability of loneliness even controlling for further variables" (p. 323). Perhaps these findings provide evidence for caution when implementing online teaching and learning, as well as other distance technology initiatives. While sometimes beneficial, online communities lack physical proximity and intimacy, potentially inhibiting opportunities for communal thanksgiving (Emmons, 2007).

Smiling and laughing can be helpful for improving mood, even when thoughts might be gloomy. Bono (2020) described a study in which participants held a pencil with either their lips (frowning) or teeth (smiling). Participants in the smiling condition were significantly more likely to rate cartoon clips as funny than were those in the frowning condition. The physical act of smiling sends signals to the brain that negative feelings may not be as bad as imagined. Neuhoff and Schaefer (2002) examined the effects of laughing, smiling, and howling on the mood of 22 adults. While howling did not have a significant impact, smiling, and to an even greater extent, laughing, both positively affected mood. Louie, Brook, and Frates (2016) stated that:

> current research is beginning to show that laughter may have serious positive physiological effects for those who engage in it on a regular basis. Providers who prescribe laughter to their patients in a structured way may be able to use these natural, free, and easily distributable positive benefits.
>
> (p. 262)

While accompanying an angry mood with excessive fake laughter might not be advisable, a gentle smile, or taking a moment to genuinely laugh off a disturbing thought, could prove beneficial.

Revisiting college professor, Paul, from the beginning of this chapter, let's consider how practicing gratitude would improve his outlook on life. Paul still teaches undergraduate and master's candidates in a rural setting, but recognizes the strength of the university within that community, and the importance of the School of Music within the campus climate. He appreciates his enthusiastic college students, and still stays in touch with many of his former K-12 students. They appreciate not only his teaching ability and knowledge, but also his positive attitude and zest for life. Paul recognizes that the mutual relationships are good for him, and keep him motivated to continue learning and seeking enriching experiences. He keeps a formal gratitude journal, listing at least three items per day, and also makes a point of internally identifying one positive fact while gently smiling or laughing, particularly during temporary moments of stress and challenge. Paul still partakes in some social media, but has limited his activity to one platform and only checks that twice per day. Instead of posting his own rants several times per day, he takes pleasure in seeing and reading other people's successes and joys. More importantly, he increases his time spent in face-to-face interactions, inviting friends for coffee, lunch, or a walk around the block with his dog. During the practice of gratitude, Paul develops an awareness that his students, colleagues, and family members are becoming more open and inviting, offering him even more opportunities for human companionship. His teaching feels easier, he starts to publish more frequently, and he fills the void of missing K-12 teaching by adjudicating, guest conducting, and offering clinics on a regular basis. Paul even embraces life in a small community, volunteering at a local dog shelter and teaching reading at a literacy bookstore. Paul is happy. Paul is grateful.

Summary

- Be aware of opportunities to give thanks.
- Consider the glass as half-full instead of half-empty. Remain positive.
- Make gratitude a habit.
- Start a gratitude journal. Writing thoughts can help to process.
- Consider long-term gratitude, including benefits from the past.
- Consider present moments of thanks. Practice mindfulness.
- Consider opportunities for future gratitude. Make a plan for thanks.
- Smile and laugh. These physical acts can help to improve mood.
- Understand why you are thankful. Dig deep to unlock reasons for gratitude.
- Turn the tide on negative news feeds and opinions of others. Recognize the good.
- When identifying headwinds (barriers), also recognize tailwinds (blessings).
- Practice gratitude alone and with others.
- Start and end every day with a moment of gratitude.

References

Algoe, S. B., Haidt, J., & Gable, S. L. (2008). Beyond reciprocity: Gratitude and relationships in everyday life. *Emotion, 8*(3), 425–429.

Bass, D. B. (2018). *Grateful: The transformative power of giving thanks*. San Francisco, CA: Harper One.

Bernhard, H. C. (2019). Gratitude, meaning, engagement, and pleasure among music educators. *New York State School Music News, 83*(1), 24–28.

Bernhard, H. C. (2020). An investigation of happiness and gratitude among music majors. *New Directions in Music Education, 4,* 1–10.

Bono, T. (2020). *Happiness 101: Simple secrets to smart living and well-being*. New York, NY: Grand Central.

Caputo, A. (2015). The relationship between gratitude and loneliness: The potential benefits of gratitude for promoting social bonds. *Europe's Journal of Psychology, 11*(2), 323–334.

Davidai, S. & Gilovich, T. (2016). The headwinds/tailwinds asymmetry: An availability bias in assessments of barriers and blessings. *Journal of Personality and Social Psychology, 111*(6), 835–851.

Elmore, T. & McPeak, A. (2019). *Generation Z unfiltered: Facing nine hidden challenges of the most anxious population*. Atlanta, GA: Poet Gardener.

Emmons, R. A. (2007). *Thanks!: How practicing gratitude can make you happier*. New York, NY: Houghton Mifflin Harcourt Publications.

Froh, J. J., Sefick, W. J., & Emmons, R. A. (2008). Counting blessings in early adolescents: An experimental study of gratitude and subjective well-being. *Journal of School Psychology, 46*(2), 213–233.

Giacalone, R. A., Paul, K., & Jurkiewicz, C. L. (2005). A preliminary investigation into the role of positive psychology in consumer sensitivity to corporate social performance. *Journal of Business Ethics, 58*(4), 295–305.

Kashdan, T. B., Mishra, A., Breen, W. E., & Froh, J. J. (2009). Gender differences in gratitude: Examining appraisals, narratives, the willingness to express emotions, and changes in psychological needs. *Journal of Personality, 77*(3), 691–730.

Kastor, D. & Hamilton, M. (2018). *Let your mind run: A memoir of thinking my way to victory*. New York, NY: Three Rivers Press.

Killen, A. & Macaskill, A. (2015). Using gratitude intervention to enhance well-being in older adults. *Journal of Happiness Studies, 16*(4), 947–964.

Lambert, N. M., Fincham, F. D., & Stillman, T. F. (2012). Gratitude and depressive symptoms: The role of positive reframing and positive emotion. *Cognition and Emotion, 26*(4), 615–633.

Louie, D., Brook, K., & Frates, E. (2016). The laughter prescription: A tool for lifestyle medicine. *American Journal of Lifestyle Medicine, 10*(4), 262–267.

McCullough, M. E., Emmons, R. A., & Tsang, J. (2002). The grateful disposition: A conceptual and empirical topography. *Journal of Personality and Social Psychology, 82,* 112–127.

Neuhoff, C. C. & Schaefer, C. (2002). Effects of laughing, smiling, and howling on mood. *Psychological Reports, 91*(3), 1079–1080.

Seligman, M. E. P. (2011). *Flourish: A visionary new understanding of happiness and well-being.* New York, NY: Simon & Schuster.
Toepfer, S. M., Cichy, K., & Peters, P. (2012). Letters of gratitude: Further evidence for author benefits. *Journal of Happiness Studies, 13,* 187–201.
Wachob, J. (2016). *Wellth: How to build a life, not a résumé.* New York, NY: Harmony Books.

6 Happiness

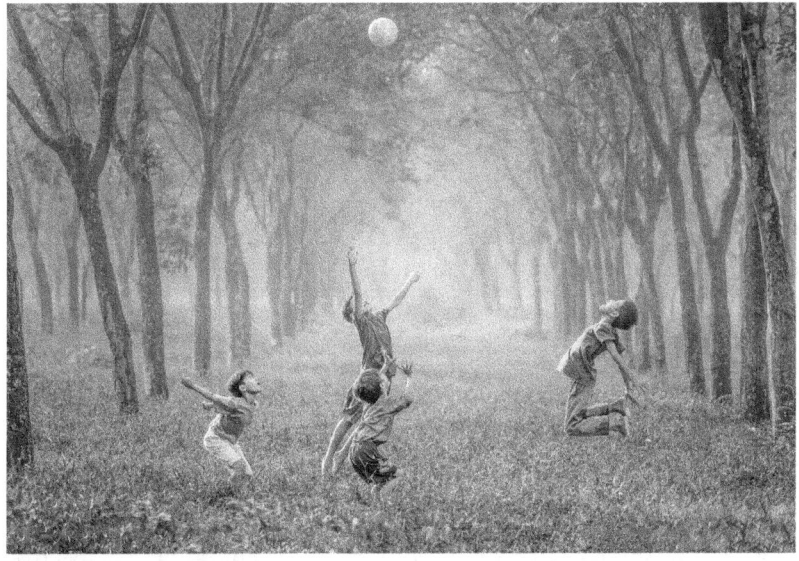

Figure 6.1 Happiness
Source: Robert Collins, Unsplash, https://unsplash.com/

Felicia feels frustrated as she watches a new set of students entering her classroom. Her administration has just added another class to her already full schedule of elementary general music. She slumps and feels defeated, realizing she doesn't even know the names of half of her 600-plus students. Felicia was a trombone music education major a few years ago, and never imagined that she would end up teaching general music. While many of her peers would be jealous of her opportunity, Felicia wishes to be anywhere but in this current situation. Instead of greeting students in the hallway between classes, Felicia scrolls through Twitter, Facebook, and Instagram feeds, longing for a return to her college days. Tough days at work multiply, and lead to sluggishness and depression after school. Friends from college and current colleagues invite Felicia to join them for meals and other entertainment, but she chooses to stay home, collapsed on her couch with the window shades drawn. She peruses smartphone advertisements for new clothing, books, and travel, but instead decides to lounge in her pajamas with a bag of chips. Her administration offers to fund conference travel and other professional development opportunities, but Felicia angrily insists that she already has a music education degree, and doesn't need further growth. Felicia feels empty and worthless.

Like college professor Paul from the previous chapter, Felicia tends to focus on negative feelings, often leading to a sense of frustrated hopelessness. "One in three adults has experienced prolonged periods of depression and one in two rate their mental health below average or poor" (Bono, 2020, p. 3). Experts from the field of positive psychology have suggested that meaning, engagement, and, to some extent, pleasure can help teachers and students manage stress and prevent burnout (e.g., Bono, 2020; Diener & Biswas-Diener, 2008; Peterson, 2018; Seligman, 2011). Peterson, Park, and Seligman (2005) defined pleasure as an immediate, hedonistic pursuit of positive sensation, meaning as long-term life purpose, and engagement as absorption in psychological flow. Thus, while "happiness" is often considered a useful life goal, more appropriate terms might be human "flourishing" or "psychological wealth." "Psychological wealth is the experience that our life is excellent – that we are living in a rewarding, engaged, meaningful, and enjoyable way" (Diener & Biswas-Diener, 2008, p. 6).

Positive psychology is not so much about being happy all the time, or a shallow sense of euphoria, but rather a balanced life perspective that leads to self-confidence, consistency, and fulfillment. In fact, in the preface to his book, Seligman (2011) wrote about his publisher's desire to place a large smiley face on the front cover. Seligman immediately resisted, concerned that readers would expect a cure-all, immediate panacea for the human condition. Bono (2020) suggested that happiness should be considered as a fluid continuum instead of a binary on or off.

> At any given point, circumstances or conditions may be beyond our control. By asking what we can do to become *happier,* we place our attention on those aspects of life that *are* in our control, which ultimately can move us forward on the happiness continuum.
>
> (p. 10)

As mentioned previously, early studies in the field of positive psychology measured pleasure, meaning, and engagement. While some researchers suggested that pleasure could be a negative quality, including hedonic pursuits that could lead to addiction and other challenges, they noted that some human pleasure is important (e.g., Seligman, 2011). For example, deep-dish pizza and chocolate cake can be nice, and even psychologically important treats on occasion, but when indulged in on a regular basis, will lead to problems. Fredrickson (2001) further studied the variable of pleasure, and suggested that positive emotion might be a more beneficial relative. She proposed a theory that experiences with positive emotion can not only help in a current moment, but can "broaden and build" psychological defense systems to help flourish in later life circumstances. By merely recalling past pleasant events, we can bring increased happiness to current situations. Fredrickson, Mancuso, Branigan, and Tugade (2000) further found that positive emotion can turn the tide on negative thoughts, which the authors coined the "undoing effect." Thus, in moments of distress, when anxious thoughts cloud our minds, we can find some relief in experiencing or recalling moments of pleasure or positive emotion.

Engagement is a psychological process of focus in which flourishing is experienced to the point that clock time seems to pass quickly and efforts feel challenging, yet satisfying (Bono, 2020; Diener & Biswas-Diener, 2008; Jackson, 2009; Seligman, 2011). Unfortunately, the human ability to concentrate in this manner seems to be deteriorating, leading to frustrated feelings of nervousness and anxiety.

> In the year 2000, the average adolescent attention span was twelve seconds ... today, the average attention span has dropped to eight seconds and the culprit seems to be social media and the Internet. One study reported that young adults between the ages of eighteen and thirty-three interact with their phones an astounding eighty-five times a day, spending several hours doing so.
> (Elmore & McPeak, 2019, p. 49)

Furthermore, Carr (2008) argued that, while the current culture of simply Googling answers in both scholarship and pop culture can be useful, it is likely leading to difficulties engaging with full-text books and articles.

Meaning is a feeling of deep life purpose. This can be experienced through long-term employment and service, or short-term opportunity, such as volunteering or offering gifts of generosity. Diener and Biswas-Diener (2008) conducted an informal experiment in which they asked college students to enjoy a hedonistic act of pleasure, such as eating ice cream, and an act of meaning, such as helping a child with homework or volunteering at a homeless shelter. Overwhelmingly, they found that most students preferred acts of meaning. While the pleasurable acts brought momentary happiness, the acts of meaning brought longer-lasting satisfaction.

> As humans, we actually require a sense of meaning to thrive. Lives that seem pointless leave us despondent and listless. We do not operate simply on instinct. We need to have values that we care about and outcomes that are worth working for.
>
> (pp. 224–225)

The Orientation to Happiness is an 18-item survey developed by Peterson, Park, and Seligman (2005) that has been employed in research studies to measure pleasure, meaning, and engagement among various populations (Table 6.1). I used the survey in two recent studies of music majors and K-12 music educators. The participants for the first study (Bernhard, 2020) were 257 music majors at a public university school of music (47.07 percent of 546 potential respondents) who were compared by year in school (freshman, sophomore, junior, senior, or graduate) and major (music education or non-music education). The secondary purpose was to examine relationships among perceived pleasure, meaning, and engagement, as well as academic/personal variables (number of credits and hours per week of classes, ensembles, homework, practice, exercise, sleep, work, and socializing). Collectively, mean scores for pleasure were comparable to university students in previous studies. Collective mean scores for engagement were lower than comparable studies, but were higher for meaning (e.g., Park, Peterson, & Ruch, 2009; Peterson, Park, & Seligman, 2005). Results of multivariate and univariate analyses of variance revealed that sophomores and juniors reported significantly higher levels of pleasure and lower levels of meaning and engagement than freshmen, seniors, or graduate students. While no significant differences in meaning or engagement were reported based on major, music education majors reported significantly lower levels of pleasure than non-music education majors. Moderate positive correlations were observed between pleasure, meaning, engagement, and reported hours of sleep.

Music education majors in this study reported lower levels of hedonic pleasure than non-music education majors, perhaps indicating some sort of connection between the teaching profession and deep life satisfaction. Further research should be pursued to determine why sophomores and juniors reported lower levels of happiness than freshmen, seniors, and graduate students. Perhaps there is a challenging

Table 6.1 Orientation to Happiness (pleasure, meaning, and engagement)

1 = not at all like me 2 = a little like me 3 = moderately like me 4 = quite a bit like me 5 = very much like me

1. Regardless of what I am doing, time passes very quickly (E).
2. My life serves a higher purpose (M).
3. Life is too short to postpone the pleasures it can provide (P).
4. I seek out situations that challenge my skills and abilities (E).
5. In choosing what to do, I always take into account whether it will benefit other people (M).
6. Whether at work or play, I am usually "in a zone" and not conscious of myself (E).
7. I am always very absorbed in what I do (E).
8. I go out of my way to feel euphoric (P).
9. In choosing what to do, I always take into account whether I can lose myself in it (E).
10. I am rarely distracted by what is going on around me (E).
11. I have a responsibility to make the world a better place (M).
12. My life has a lasting meaning (M).
13. In choosing what to do, I always take into account whether it will be pleasurable (P).
14. What I do matters to society (M).
15. I agree with this statement: "Life is short – eat dessert first" (P).
16. I love to do things that excite my senses (P).
17. I have spent a lot of time thinking about what life means and how I fit into its big picture (M).
18. For me, the good life is the pleasurable life (P).

Source: Peterson, Park, and Seligman (2005)

point in undergraduate music study, when the excitement of freshman year has worn off, and a light at the end of the tunnel is still too distant. Further study should also be pursued to determine why collective scores for engagement were so low. One possible explanation could be related to the current culture of digital distraction. As Jackson (2009) argued, "The way we live is eroding our capacity for deep, sustained, perceptive attention – the building block of intimacy, wisdom, and cultural progress" (p. 13). However, collective scores for meaning were relatively strong, as were positive correlations between happiness and hours of sleep.

The participants for the second study (Bernhard, 2019) were 235 music teachers from the state of New York (47 percent of 500 potential respondents) who were compared by grade level taught (elementary, middle, high school, or a combination), certification status (initial or professional), and teaching area (instrumental, choral/general, or a combination). The secondary purpose was to examine relationships among perceived pleasure, meaning, and engagement, as well as teaching/personal variables (number of hours per week of teaching, preparing, exercising, sleeping, socializing, family obligations, and working another job). Collectively, mean scores for pleasure were comparable to adults in previous studies. Collective mean scores for engagement were slightly lower than comparable studies, but were higher for meaning (e.g., Giacalone, Paul, & Jurkiewicz, 2005; Park, Peterson, & Ruch, 2009; Peterson, Park, & Seligman, 2005). Results of multivariate and univariate analyses of variance revealed that elementary school teachers reported higher levels of meaning and pleasure than others, and high school teachers reported higher levels of engagement than others. While no significant differences in pleasure or engagement were reported based on certification status, early career teachers (four or fewer years in the profession) reported lower levels of meaning than those with more experience. Regarding teaching area, no significant differences were found regarding pleasure, but instrumental teachers and those who teach in a combination of areas reported higher levels of meaning and engagement than those in the choral/general music category. Moderate positive correlations were observed between meaning, engagement, and reported hours of teaching and exercise. Moderate negative correlations were observed among reported hours of teaching and hours of sleep.

Collectively, music teachers in this study reported relatively healthy levels of pleasure, meaning, and engagement compared to previous literature with adult participants, perhaps indicating a connection between the music teaching profession and life satisfaction. Further research should be pursued to determine why middle school teachers and those in choral/general music settings reported lower levels of meaning and engagement than their peers. Support should also continue for new teachers, who, as in previous literature, reported greater challenges than those with more experience.

Recommendations for Practicing Happiness

As with gratitude, one of the first steps in practicing happiness is developing awareness of positive emotion. Remember that the point is not to be swinging from emotional highs to lows on a regular basis, but to develop a regular sense of fulfillment and vitality. When identifying positive emotions, take care to avoid undue comparisons with others. "We naturally compare ourselves with those around us ... and with others' circumstances as our barometer, we can be led to make decisions that are *objectively* worse for us so long as they are *relatively* better than someone else's" (Bono, 2020, p. 32). In a classic study by Tversky and Griffin (1991), the researchers asked undergraduate students to predict their own happiness regarding hypothetical salaries in a new job. The first scenario offered the new employees $35,000 per year while their comparable peers made $38,000. The second scenario offered only $33,000 per year, with comparable peers being paid $30,000. While the majority of students opted for the higher paying offer, they predicted that they would be happier in the second scenario. More recently, social media has created a challenging culture in which comparison is difficult to avoid. Viewing the seemingly perfect lives of others, or perhaps comparing the number of likes, shares, and retweets, can cause undue stress and negative emotion. "No matter how good you are at something, or how you rank your accomplishments, there is someone out there who makes you look incompetent … compare yourself to who you were yesterday, not to who someone else is today" (Peterson, 2018, p. 85).

Avoiding or minimizing comparisons with others is a good start, but negative emotions will occur at some point for all of us. "We are hardwired to give more attention to the bad than the good" (Bono, 2020, p. 198). In these moments, resilience and rebounding are important factors for once again experiencing positive emotion and leading to deeper life meaning. Elmore and McPeak (2019) encouraged practices of growth mindset, hope, visual aids, and autonomy to aid resilience and development of meaning. Growth mindset was coined by Carol Dweck, and works in contrast to fixed mindset. "With this mindset, people acknowledge that effort and hard work are necessary for success" (Bono, 2020, p. 140). Similarly, the concept of hope suggests that we are able to learn new ideas and move forward from hardships. Visual aids work to accompany verbal information and are often processed more easily. "We're incredible at remembering pictures. Hear a piece of information, and three days later you'll remember 10 percent of it. Add a picture and you'll remember 65 percent" (Medina Brain Rules, 2020). Autonomy, or control, allows individuals empowerment to shift from negative to positive emotions, and to develop deeper levels of life meaning (Elmore & McPeak, 2019).

As mentioned earlier in this chapter, the ability to engage and stay focused is an important component of happiness and life satisfaction, yet it is more easily stated than done. Positive psychologists and other researchers have posited that engagement is particularly challenging in the current culture of smart technology. "We may have sat down at our desks to work on a project or begin an important paper, but our automatic impulses quickly draw us into our favorite social media sites" (Bono, 2020, p. 100). "Human satisfaction is shifting. We are more and more content with a virtual experience, instead of a real one" (Elmore & McPeak, 2019, p. 64).

Sciandra and Inman (2016) examined the impacts of smartphones on the shopping habits of consumers from around the United States. While they found the technology can be helpful in making decisions and saving money, using bar-code scanning apps and digital coupons, they also demonstrated that deleterious effects of digital distraction were present. Shopping interruptions for consumers to check email, text messages, and social media caused many to take extra time, or even forget some planned purchases. Kushlev, Proulx, and Dunn (2016) studied the impact of digital distraction via smartphone notification alerts. Two hundred and twenty-one adult participants were instructed to spend one week with smartphones nearby with notification alerts enabled, followed by another week with smartphones tucked away and notification alerts disabled. "Participants reported higher levels of inattention and hyperactivity when alerts were on than when alerts were off. Higher levels of inattention in turn predicted lower productivity and psychological well-being" (p. 1011).

In addition to the mindfulness exercises presented later in this book, psychologists have suggested limiting digital interaction and reframing sources of motivation. Disabling smartphone notifications and removing social media apps can minimize the temptation to check email, text messages, and newsfeeds on an excessive basis. Ironically, smart-apps such as "Forest" can help users stay focused by setting timers and growing virtual trees during time engaged in work. Bono (2020) recommended dividing large projects into smaller chunks, moving through gradual steps to a larger final goal. For example, awarding small pieces of candy when various points of a hardcopy book have been reached can allow readers to enjoy small treats as they move through complex ideas. He also suggested that deadlines be considered beneficial instead of problematic. By setting several short deadlines within the timeframe of a long-term project, motivation and happiness can be increased. "You might think that having more time is always better, but sometimes having *less* time is what serves us best of all. Tight deadlines prompt high-quality work, and limited time leads us to savor an experience more" (Bono, 2020, p. 171).

Recently, positive psychologists have added the importance of human relationships and personal accomplishments to the variables of pleasure/positive emotion, meaning, and engagement. As discussed in Chapter 5 in this book about gratitude, joining fellow human beings in thanksgiving or other activities can help to combat feelings of isolation and loneliness. In-person human interaction is particularly important in the current digital climate. Lloyd (2010) cautioned readers to consider the potential dangers of online interactions. "There is a 'reality' to being online which we know to be false. We are simultaneously 'there' but 'not there' as we talk, work and play with others in online spaces" (p. 1). Elsobeihi and Abu Naser (2017) studied the impact of mobile device use on the quantity and quality of face-to-face interaction among university students. Not surprisingly, they found that both the quantity and the quality of human relationships had been negatively impacted by technology.

To combat these challenges, Elmore and McPeak (2019) recommended limiting the number of social media accounts and time spent in such environments.

> The irony of social media use is that it is both self-soothing and a source of anxiety ... we often resort to it when we don't know what to do with ourselves, yet it frequently becomes a root cause of negative emotions: angst, envy, and the fear of missing out.
>
> (p. 150)

Bono (2020) reinforced the importance of face-to-face relationships. "High-quality friendships provide a support structure during life's challenges, along with a means of helping us celebrate life's joys ... and provide a buffer against physical ailments" (p. 218). Bono further explained that life experiences with others usually bring greater happiness than material purchases or possessions. Anticipating upcoming travel and other experiences can be as pleasurable as the actual moment, as can positive reminiscence following the occasion.

Personal accomplishment has long been a component of burnout measures, with perceived lack of accomplishment correlating strongly with feelings of emotional exhaustion and depersonalization (e.g., Maslach, Jackson, & Schwab, 1986), but has more recently been considered an important variable in the field of positive psychology (e.g., Bono, 2020; Elmore & McPeak, 2019; Peterson, 2018; Wachob, 2016). Recognition of personal accomplishments can lead to feelings of satisfaction, confidence, and self-esteem. They can also lead to strong feelings of self-efficacy, improving the chances of further accomplishments. Peterson (2018) wrote that even body posture can impact self-confidence and accomplishment, resulting in changing levels of serotonin. "Low serotonin means decreased confidence ... low serotonin means less happiness, more pain and anxiety, more illness, and a shorter lifespan" (p. 15). Similarly, Brinol, Petty, and Wagner (2009) examined the effects of body posture on self-evaluations of adults and found that sitting erect with chest pushed out led to more confident evaluations than when slouching forward with backs curved.

Bono (2020) suggested that self-efficacy can be improved through prior accomplishment, particularly when that accomplishment involves offering help to others. "When we accomplish one task, we become confident that we can accomplish other tasks. The narrow time window that once felt overwhelming suddenly becomes more manageable" (p. 187). Elmore and McPeak (2019) supported this notion, but warned that working hard toward accomplishment should not be confused with entitlement. Receiving benefits without effort, or perceiving that one is entitled to benefits without effort, will ultimately lead to feelings of disappointment. Rather, it is important to embrace a growth mindset and develop what Duckworth (2016) coined as "grit," perseverance and passion for long-term goals.

Revisiting general music teacher, Felicia, from the beginning of this chapter, let's consider how practices related to happiness and positive psychology would improve her outlook on life. Felicia stands in the hallway, enthusiastically greeting a new class of elementary school students as they enter her music room. She sings a short tune that incorporates the names of each student, and they echo with enjoyment. Felicia is recovering from a mild cold, but ate and slept well the night before, and now savors some herbal tea as she moves through the school day. During brief moments of fatigue, she reminds herself to stand tall and breathe deeply. She turns her smartphone off throughout the school day, and uses it minimally while at home, instead choosing to read more about general music teaching methodologies, taking care of herself, and spending time with close friends. One of the books Felicia reads leads to an awareness of an upcoming professional conference, which her administration is happy to fund. During discussions related to conference travel, Felicia is able to explain to her administration that her teaching would be enhanced with one less class and an extra few minutes per section. She volunteers to serve on a scheduling committee the following summer, and makes initial strides toward a more reasonable teaching load and the hiring of a new colleague. Felicia laughs when reflecting on how much she despised general music as a trombone major in college. She finds deep meaning in her work, and wouldn't want life to be any different. Felicia's friends, colleagues, and students love spending time with her, and the following year she is recognized as her school's teacher of the year.

Summary

- Be aware of opportunities for positive emotion.
- Consider the glass as half-full instead of half-empty. Turn the tide on negative emotion.
- Treat comparisons with caution.
- Avoid digital and other forms of distraction. Engage deeply.
- Limit social media and disable smartphone notifications.

- Embrace in-person relationships with others.
- Stand tall. Look confident to feel confident.
- Recognize opportunities for deep meaning.
- Recognize and celebrate accomplishments.
- Learn from failures and rebound readily.

References

Bernhard, H. C. (2019). Gratitude, meaning, engagement, and pleasure among music educators. *New York State School Music News, 83*(1), 24–28.

Bernhard, H. C. (2020). An investigation of happiness and gratitude among music majors. *New Directions in Music Education, 4,* 1–10.

Bono, T. (2020). *Happiness 101: Simple secrets to smart living and well-being.* New York, NY: Grand Central.

Brinol, P., Petty, R. E., & Wagner, B. (2009). Body posture effects on self-evaluation: A self-validation approach. *European Journal of Social Psychology, 39*(6), 1053–1064.

Carr, N. (2008). Is Googling making us stupid? *The Atlantic.* July/August.

Diener, E. & Biswas-Diener, R. (2008). *Happiness: Unlocking the mysteries of psychological wealth.* Malden, MA: Blackwell.

Duckworth, A. (2016). *Grit: The power of passion and perseverance.* New York, NY: Scribner.

Elmore, T. & McPeak, A. (2019). *Generation Z unfiltered: Facing nine hidden challenges of the most anxious population.* Atlanta, GA: Poet Gardener.

Elsobeihi, M. M. & Abu Naser, S. S. (2017). Effects of mobile technology on human relationships. *International Journal of Engineering and Information Systems, 1*(5), 110–125.

Fredrickson, B. L. (2001). The role of positive emotions in positive psychology: The broaden-and-build theory of positive emotions. *American Psychologist, 56,* 218–226.

Fredrickson, B. L., Mancuso, R. A., Branigan, C., & Tugade, M. M. (2000). The undoing effect of positive emotions. *Motivation and Emotion, 24,* 237–258.

Giacalone, R. A., Paul, K., & Jurkiewicz, C. L. (2005). A preliminary investigation into the role of positive psychology in consumer sensitivity to corporate social performance. *Journal of Business Ethics, 58*(4), 295–305.

Jackson, M. (2009). *Distracted: The erosion of attention and the coming dark age.* Amherst, NY: Prometheus Books.

Kushlev, K., Proulx, J., & Dunn, E. W. (2016). "Silence your phones": Smartphone notifications increase inattention and hyperactivity symptoms. *CHI '16: Proceedings of the 2016 CHI Conference on Human Factors in Computing Systems,* 1011–1020.

Lloyd, M. (2010). There, yet not there: Human relationships with technology. *Journal of Learning Design, 3*(2), 1–13.

Maslach, C., Jackson, S. E., & Schwab, R. L. (1986). *Maslach Burnout Inventory – Educators Survey.* Palo Alto, CA: College of California, Consulting Psychologists Press.

Medina Brain Rules. (2020). Retrieved February 1, 2020, from www.brainrules.net/vision

Park, N., Peterson, C., & Ruch, W. (2009). Orientation to happiness and life satisfaction in twenty-seven nations. *Journal of Positive Psychology, 4*(4), 273–279.

Peterson, C., Park, N., & Seligman, M. E. P. (2005). Orientation to happiness and life satisfaction: The full life versus the empty life. *Journal of Happiness Studies, 6*, 25–41.

Peterson, J. B. (2018). *12 rules for life: An antidote to chaos*. Toronto, ON: Random House Canada.

Seligman, M. E. P. (2011). *Flourish: A visionary new understanding of happiness and well-being*. New York, NY: Simon & Schuster.

Sciandra, M. & Inman, J. (2016). Digital distraction: Consumer mobile device use and decision making. Retrieved February 1, 2020, from: https://ssrn.com/abstract=2439202

Tversky, A. & Griffin, D. (1991). Endowment and contrast judgements of well-being. In R. J. Zeckhauser (Ed.), *Strategy and choice* (p. 313). Cambridge, MA: MIT Press.

Wachob, J. (2016). *Wellth: How to build a life, not a résumé*. New York, NY: Harmony Books.

7 Mindfulness

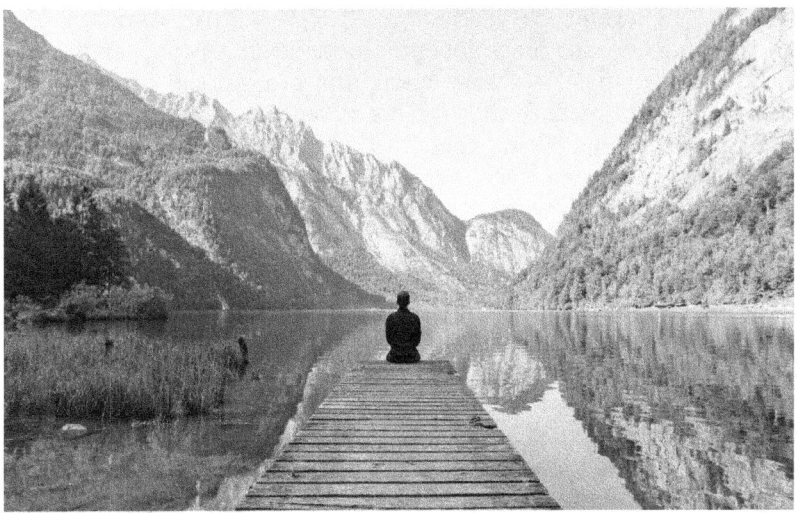

Figure 7.1 Mindfulness
Source: Simon Migaj, Unsplash, https://unsplash.com/

Amy races from her car into the school building. She overslept her alarm again, slammed down a fast-food croissant and coffee while speeding to work, and now feels flustered as she runs to first period orchestra rehearsal, arriving at the same time as her students. She didn't sleep well the previous night, worrying about whether her students will make it through all five pieces of an upcoming concert (and realizing she forgot to prepare a printed program or arrange for custodial services). Amy also lets her mind wander to the past, lamenting the loss of several strong seniors from the previous year. If only they could help drown out the sounds of her weaker players, she thinks, all would be okay. Her mind continues to spin as students stumble into rehearsal. She can't figure out whether to start with announcements, tuning, or collecting money from a current fundraiser. Amy struggles to breathe as she rummages through her briefcase and starts barking orders for the beginning of another frantic day.

If reading this vignette causes physical tension in your body, you can now take a deep breath and consider the potential benefits of mindfulness practice. While mindfulness, or what is also known as contemplative practice, is sometimes considered spiritual, touchy-feely, or too close to formal religion, current secular practices are gaining support for general use in society, including education (e.g., Berg & Seeber, 2016; Hall, 2015; Hawkins, 2017; Jennings, 2015; Nel, 2014; Varona, 2018). These researchers and practitioners have studied the use of mindfulness in teacher training, K-12 instruction, and professional development. Srinivasan (2014) defined mindfulness as "energy we cultivate through kind, present-moment awareness" (p. 27). Kahn (2019) added that mindfulness involves a level of curiosity and non-judgment, observing thoughts and actions without assigning formal assessment. It involves recognition of the present, inhabiting the physical body and recognizing current surroundings. Reflections about the past and plans for the future are certainly necessary and good, but excessive mental rumination can become problematic. While formal diagnoses of depression and anxiety are complex and beyond the scope of this book, a general starting point can be described as depression linked to excessive regrets about missing or wanting to change the past, and anxiety linked to excessive worry about what might happen in the future. Recognizing that we can only truly control the present moment allows for a slowing of pace and awareness of current feelings, physical sensations, and actions (e.g., Holzel et al., 2011; Tang et al., 2007).

Mindfulness can help to alleviate excessive worry, or what is sometimes known as "catastrophizing." Consider the number of times you worry about a potential future problem, only to later realize that the issue never materialized. Again, a calm level of planning is important, but excessive worry about that which cannot be controlled is problematic. Similarly, it is challenging to ruminate excessively about past experiences, none of which can be relived. While healthy reflection and learning from past successes and mistakes are good, living in the past, whether wishing it had been different or wanting a return to past glory days, will lead to disappointment. In the opening vignette, orchestra teacher Amy catastrophizes about potential challenges to successfully performing five pieces in an upcoming concert, leading to problems in other areas of teaching and her personal life. She fails to slow her pace, recognize shallow breathing and other physical tensions, and consider healthy options for moving forward. By starting with proper care of herself, including a good night's sleep, Amy will be in a better position to calmly address one issue at a time before, during, and after rehearsal. Her focus on past students and successes also hinders Amy's ability to focus on current students, perhaps including the selection of a more reasonable repertoire and more realistic goals for fundraising and other administrative tasks.

Mindfulness-Based-Stress-Reduction (MBSR) is a widely known program developed by Jon Kabat-Zinn and taught by many around the world. The following are nine goals of the program, with accompanying descriptions (Kahn, 2019).

1. *Non-judging* – Assume the stance of an impartial witness to your own experience. Cultivate discernment; recognizing and understanding what is actually happening and unfolding, without judgement.
2. *Patience* – This is a form of wisdom. It demonstrates that we understand and accept the fact that sometimes things must unfold in their own time. When we are present with ourselves, we inhabit the present moment with acceptance.
3. *Beginner's Mind* – A mind willing to see everything as if for the first time. In the expert mind there are few possibilities, in the mind of the beginner, infinite possibilities.
4. *Trust* – Trust yourself and your own basic wisdom and goodness. Trust in the practice.
5. *Non-striving* – Simply allow anything and everything that we experience from moment to moment to be here, because it already is. In doing so, we bring a much greater wisdom and appropriateness to our experience.
6. *Acceptance* – This is a willingness to see things as they actually are. An active recognition, an acknowledgement of what is unfolding before us. A reality check, without judgement or analyzation.
7. *Letting Go* – This is a way of letting things be, of accepting things as they are. We let them be, and in doing so, we let them go.
8. *Generosity* – Do something for someone for its own sake, not to get anything in return.
9. *Gratitude* – Start and end your day with a moment of gratitude. Acknowledge all you have for which to be grateful.

These nine goals are addressed through both formal and informal mindfulness practices. Two types of formal practice can be particularly useful for teachers; breathing meditation and body scan. Breathing meditation involves taking time to focus on the inhalation and exhalation of breath. While thoughts will likely surface during this process, it is important to simply observe those ideas, without judgment. Thoughts, whether positive, negative, or neutral, should be noticed without labeling.

> Close your eyes. Pay attention to your breathing and see whether you can find the place in your body where you most clearly feel the sensations of your breath moving in and out. You might notice it at the tip of your nose or in the rise and fall of your belly or chest. It makes no difference at all where you feel your breath; there's no "right" place. Now just let your attention settle on that place, and watch your breath as it moves in and back out. With an attitude of relaxed curiosity, count ten breaths. Don't try to change or control your breathing. You don't need to do any special or fancy breathing. Just count ten inhalations and ten exhalations. You may notice that your mind wanders quickly, maybe even before the end of the first breath. When that happens, without judging yourself or your wandering mind, bring your attention back to your breath. Stop after you've completed ten breaths.
> (Rogers, 2016, pp. 22–23)

Similarly, body scan is a formal practice that involves focusing on specific parts of the physical self, without judgment. Instead, calm awareness of feelings, whether tense, loose, or neutral, allow space for slowing of pace and recognition of physical sensations.

> Begin by bringing awareness to the bottoms of your feet as you notice the feeling of your feet resting against the floor. Perhaps you notice pressure where your feet make contact with the floor, or the touch of your socks on your skin. Maybe you notice tingling or other sensations, or maybe you don't notice much sensation at all. It makes no difference; you are not trying to change anything, just to see what is actually happening in this moment. As you continue to watch the sensations in your feet, allow yourself to become aware of your breath moving in and out of your body. If it seems helpful, try to imagine your breath moving in and out through the bottoms of your feet. With each in-breath, allow your awareness to sharpen; with each out-breath, allow tension and tightness to be released from your feet. Breathing in, focus your attention; breathing out, release tension. After a minute or so, move your awareness up to your lower legs. With an attitude of curiosity, see whether you notice any sensations in your

shins or calf muscles. Can you feel your pants or socks touching your skin? Do you notice pulsations or tingles in your legs? Can you notice the muscles in your legs? Begin to imagine your breath moving in and out through your calf muscles, and with each in-breath sharpen your focus on the sensations; with each out-breath release tightness and tension. If your mind wanders, see whether you are able to notice that your attention has shifted, without judging yourself. You are seeing the nature of your mind at its most clear and natural when you observe the way your mind shifts, producing thoughts moving from one topic to the next. Bring your attention back to the sensations in your lower legs. After a minute or so, move your attention to your upper legs, your thighs. Again notice whatever sensations are present, and if it is helpful, imagine your breathing moving in and out through the muscles of your thighs, releasing tightness and tension as you exhale, focusing your awareness as you inhale. Continue moving slowly up the body in this manner, spending a few minutes on various body parts. After your upper legs, you can notice your hands on your lap, your arms, your back and shoulders, your neck, your jaw, the muscles around your eyes, and your forehead. Depending on how much time you wish to spend meditating, you can visit fewer or more places, spending just a few minutes at each spot, breathing in and out and noticing the sensations. Before you finish, take a few moments to slowly scan your awareness through your body from head to toe. If you notice any areas of tightness or tension, let your awareness settle there for a few moments, breathing in and out through that tight place, and observing the sensations there. And again, when you notice your mind has wandered, just observe that. Allow yourself to be a curious scientist learning about how thoughts flow, rather than a punitive prison guard flogging yourself for moving outside the box. Finally, settle your attention on your breath, watching the sensations as you take two or three slow, deep breaths before opening your eyes. Take a few moments to stretch in any way that feels comfortable before getting up.

(Rogers, 2016, pp. 38–39)

While regular practice of these formal meditations can be an important part of developing mindfulness, the more useful long-term outcome involves informal awareness throughout a given day. This can be particularly important for teachers, as it allows space to notice what is truly happening in any given moment; to see, hear, feel, and otherwise sense the present moment. While this, again, might seem overly spiritual, the goal of secular mindfulness is simply to notice when tensions might be mounting, or when thoughts and decision-making processes are becoming cluttered. By taking a step back, even for a few seconds, it becomes possible to gently assess the current situation and make objective decisions that will ultimately reduce stress and tension (e.g., Birnie, Speca, & Carlson, 2010; Mindfulness and Health, 2016).

A particularly useful form of informal mindfulness practice for music teachers involves that of listening. As we interact with the psychological properties of pitch, rhythm, timbre, and loudness, and rehearse for intonation, tone quality, articulation, precision, phrasing, balance and blend, etc., it is imperative that we sharpen listening acuity. Mindfulness practices offer an opportunity to deepen listening skills, for both music and spoken language. According to Barbezat and Bush (2014), "deep listening is a way of hearing in which we are fully present with what is happening in the moment ... very few have developed this capacity for listening" (p. 137). Similarly, Treasure (2011) warned that most humans do not fully listen, and are even likely to purposefully ignore incoming aural stimuli. Experts from the Listening Center (2019) stated that humans spend approximately half of their time listening, but are distracted or forgetful about 75 percent of that time.

To counteract these challenges, university professors associated with the Center for Contemplative Mind in Society (2019) incorporated best practice listening activities into topics including chemistry, law, and architecture. At Bryn Mawr College, for example, chemistry students were instructed to:

> start with the sounds closest to you ... the pumps chugging at the lab bench, the roar of the fume hoods. Slowly extend your awareness outward in circles. Let go of thoughts and emotions and return to the simple sound.

Similarly, Boorstein (1996) compared radars that send information with satellite dishes that receive, suggesting that we are more like satellite dishes; powered on and ready to receive, but quiet and waiting (Center for Contemplative Mind in Society, 2019).

In music education, these suggestions can easily correspond to rehearsal settings and classes, both as ensemble member and leader. For example, students should be encouraged to listen specifically for bass lines, melodies, or harmonies, close their eyes to listen for those singing or playing the same part, or simply attend to silence occurring within a given musical excerpt. These exercises can be extended to other aspects of life, listening for weather patterns while walking outside, listening for mechanical sounds while inside, and listening with focused purpose while engaged in conversation with others.

In addition to these listening activities, mindfulness can be used with students to encourage focus and compassion (Hawkins, 2017; Jennings, 2015; Srinivasan 2014). During classes or rehearsals, consider using the aforementioned breathing or body scan activities, even for short periods of time. Calm, relaxed breathing can help to quiet and focus students, while also positively contributing to air circulation for singers and wind instrumentalists. Similarly, body awareness can contribute positively to physical warm-ups, easing into neuromusculoskelatal health. Compassion meditation is another traditional mindfulness activity, and one that can work particularly well with students. The activity involves breathing meditation with periods of time to focus on gratitude and well wishes for ourselves, those we already love, those we may not know very well, and those who challenge us in daily life.

> Take three deep breaths. Your breath helps you create awareness of what is happening in the here and now. Your breath can also help you calm yourself. Once you calm yourself down you'll know that you are ultimately okay and that whatever you are facing is workable. We need to be able to accept whatever we are experiencing. Once you feel better you can observe the emotion while it is happening. Naming the emotion can help it feel less overwhelming. "I'm feeling anger right now." Whatever the emotion is, try to experience it fully. Don't judge it. There's nothing wrong with it. Once you have labeled and accepted the emotion as it is, ask yourself, "What do I feel in my body? Why is this emotion there?" Using your breath, hold yourself with love. Be kind to yourself when you experience a challenging emotion. If it is still too overwhelming, try to turn your attention to your breath. You are not trying to ignore your emotion; you are trying to see it clearly. Through clearly seeing your emotion you will take it less personally. Inside we have all kinds of seeds. All the time we are watering seeds, but we can build mindfulness and try to water the helpful seeds in ourselves and others more than the unhelpful seeds. Mindfulness helps us become aware of what seeds we are watering.
>
> (Srinivasan, 2014, pp. 196–197)

Mindfulness has also been used effectively in higher education. Tang et al., (2007) studied the effects of short-term meditation practices on the attention and self-regulation of Chinese undergraduate students. Eighty students participated, half of whom received five days of 20-minute meditation sessions. The meditation treatment promoted a restful state of alertness with attention to body, breathing, and external instructions from a compact disc player. "Because this approach is suitable for novices, we hypothesized that a short period of training and practice might influence the efficiency of the executive attention network related to self-regulation" (p. 17153). Participants from this experimental group reported reduced anxiety, depression, anger, and fatigue, as well as lowered stress-related cortisol levels as compared to control group participants.

Shapiro, Schwartz, and Bonner (1998) tested the effects of eight weeks of mindfulness-based stress reduction intervention instruction on the mental health of medical students. They defined mindfulness-based stress reduction (MBSR) as a formal discipline including meditation, that promotes heightened awareness with a focus on compassion for self and others. Following treatment for 37 experimental group participants, the researchers reported that MBSR can effectively "(1) reduce self-reports of overall psychological distress including depression, (2) reduce self-reported state and trait anxiety, (3) increase scores on overall empathy levels, and (4) increase scores on a measure of spiritual experiences assessed at termination of the intervention" (p. 592).

In a more recent study, Shapiro, Brown, and Biegel (2007) studied the effects of MBSR on the mental health of student therapists. The participants were 64 master's students enrolled at a small private Jesuit university (22 received treatment and 42 served as control, based on enrollment in three graduate courses). The MBSR treatment occurred over the course of eight weeks, two hours per week, and as with the previous study, included heightened awareness via meditation with a focus on compassion for self and others. The researchers found that MBSR reduced stress, negative affect, rumination, and anxiety, while increasing positive affect and self-compassion. Findings from these studies suggest that meditation may be useful in the interpersonal health and psychological well-being of pre-professionals who are training to help other humans.

Meditation via MBSR has also been used to improve intrapersonal feelings. Birnie, Speca, and Carlson (2010) examined the use of MBSR in a community setting (participants were volunteers from Fall 2005 until Spring 2007 in a program offered to the public through the University of Calgary), and found that it positively influenced kindness toward oneself, perceptions of connection, and a balance of internal thoughts, such that negativity did not predominate. Holzel et al., (2011) reviewed neuroimaging studies that demonstrated how meditation can cause neuroplastic changes in the brain, such that participants positively alter how they identify and conceive of themselves. They stated that "these changes occur in the anterior cingulate cortex, insula, temporo-parietal junction, fronto-limbic network, and default mode network structures" (p. 537), which can improve self-perception, well-being, and cognitive functioning. Using similar neuroimaging evidence, Immordino-Yang and Damasio (2008) suggested that these types of intrapersonal exploration are important in the development of the emotional responses needed for effective teaching and learning.

Mindfulness is a natural partner with other parts of this book. For example, difficulties with sleep can sometimes be negotiated through mindful breathing. If you're having trouble falling asleep or are wake for extended periods of time during the night, try the breathing or body scan activities previously described. Both can help to avoid judgmental focus on thoughts and associated worry about past or future events.

> Breathe through your nose for about two seconds, with your belly moving outward more than your chest. As you breathe out, gently press your belly, which will push up on your diaphragm and help you get air out. Repeat until you feel yourself getting sleepy.
>
> (Migala, 2019, p. 31)

Mindful eating can help to slow the pace of food consumption, leading to better dietary choices and healthier mealtime experiences. Instead of gorging food while watching a ten-minute clip of Food Network's *Diners, Drive-ins, and Dives,* turn away from technology and take time to savor each bite of nutrition. "Mindful eating –taking time to experience the taste, texture, look and smell of food – helps us gauge how much we're consuming while keeping us in touch with our internal hunger cues" (Goldman, 2019, p. 94). Finally, physical movement can be enhanced through mindfulness, taking time to relax and feel each gentle expression of the human form. Moving around a classroom or through a school building can become a more relaxed and purposeful activity by mindfully becoming aware of how each footstep feels, and taking time to appreciate the current physical and psychological space.

> Exercise is one of the best ways to deflect the stress of the workday, and you can get physical and emotional benefits just from walking. Even a 15-minute walk helps people focus more at work and feel less exhausted at the end of the day.
>
> (MacMillan, 2019, p. 78)

Using suggestions from this chapter, let's now revisit orchestra teacher, Amy, from a more mindful perspective. Amy walks slowly, yet purposefully, into the school building. She savored her commute to school, enjoying a beautiful sunrise and noticing other people around her. She slept soundly the night before, even though she woke early to eat a nutritious breakfast and mindfully read the newspaper. Although her schedule didn't allow for a formal meditation session, she ran a slow mile around her neighborhood before showering and getting ready for the day. Upon entering the school building, Amy notices the quiet in her steps as she walks to retrieve programs for the upcoming concert. She reflects about how this event will be different from last year, including more chamber music than full orchestra works, which will allow heterogeneous ability levels to be properly showcased among her current group of diverse students. Without judging for better or worse, Amy takes a deep and confident breath, and begins greeting students who are also making their way to the orchestra rehearsal room. Some of the students ask about fundraising accounts, but Amy simply reminds them that a parent is now in charge of those funds, and that the money will be collected every Friday morning. Upon arrival at the room, Amy is pleased to notice that several students are already helping each other tune instruments, and starting the process of warming-up in small groups. She projects a computer image of announcements for the day and takes another deep breath before calmly making her way around the room to finish coaching students for the upcoming concert.

Summary

- Be aware of the present moment. Savor it.
- Focus on the breath, noticing passing thoughts without judgment.
- Be aware of physical sensation. If tense, breathe and observe.
- Embrace learning. Acknowledge that it's okay to not know.
- Remember the past, and learn from it, but do not dwell on it.
- Plan for the future, with calm mind, but do not panic.
- Forgive, others and yourself.
- Be generous, to others and yourself.
- Be patient, with others and yourself.

References

Barbezat, D. P., & Bush, M. (2014). *Contemplative practices in higher education: Powerful methods to transform teaching and learning.* San Francisco, CA: Jossey-Bass.

Berg, M., & Seeber, B. K. (2016). *The slow professor: Challenging the culture of speed in the academy.* Toronto, ON: University of Toronto Press.

Birnie, K., Speca, M., & Carlson, L. E. (2010). Exploring self-compassion and empathy in the context of mindfulness-based stress reduction (MBSR). *Stress and Health, 26*(5), 359–371.

Boorstein, S. (1996). *Don't just do something; sit there.* San Francisco, CA: Harper One.

Center for Contemplative Mind in Society. (2019). Retrieved May 15, 2019, from www.contemplativemind.org/programs/acmhe

Goldman, L. (2019). Trending: Body kindness. In L. Lombardi (Ed.). *TIME special edition: The new mindfulness* (pp. 92–94). New York, NY: Meredith Corporation.

Hall, C. (2015). *Is your brain being Googled to death?* Retrieved May 21, 2019, from www.dallasnews.com/business/columnists/cheryl-hall/20151117-is-your-brain-being-googled-to-death.ece

Hawkins, K. (2017). *Mindful teacher, mindful school: Improving wellbeing in teaching and learning.* Thousand Oaks, CA: Sage.

Holzel, B. K., Lazar, S. W., Gard, T., Schuman-Olivier, Z., Vago, D. R., & Ott, U. (2011). How does mindfulness meditation work? Proposing mechanisms of action from a conceptual and neural perspective. *Perspectives on Psychological Science, 6*(6), 537–559.

Immordino-Yang, M. H., & Damasio, A. (2008). We feel, therefore we learn: The relevance of affective and social neuroscience to education. In M. H. Immordino-Yang (Ed.), *The Jossey-Bass reader on the brain and learning* (pp. 183–198). San Francisco, CA: Jossey-Bass.

Jennings, P. A. (2015). *Mindfulness for teachers: Simple skills for peace and productivity in the classroom.* New York, NY: W. W. Norton.

Kahn, M. (2019). Retrieved June 1, 2019, from https://www.mindfulnesstrainingsrc.com/

Listening Center. (2019). Retrieved May 27, 2019, from http://sacredlistening.com/tlc_listening101.htm

MacMillan, J. (2019). 6 more reasons to get up and move. In L. Lombardi (Ed.). *TIME special edition: The new mindfulness* (pp. 76–79). New York, NY: Meredith Corporation.

Migala, J. (2019). 13 ways breathing better improves your life. In L. Lombardi (Ed.). *TIME special edition: The new mindfulness* (pp. 28–31). New York, NY: Meredith Corporation.

Mindfulness and Health: A Multidisciplinary Scholarly Conference. (2016). Retrieved May 22, 2019, from www.wnycollegeconnection.com/documents/contemplative

Nel, P. (2014). *In search of lost time: Why faculty members work so much.* Retrieved May 23, 2019 from https://www.insidehighered.com/advice/2014/03/03/essay-why-faculty-members-work-so-much

Rogers, H. B. (2016). *The mindful twenty-something: Life skills to handle stress and everything else.* Oakland, CA: New Harbinger Publications.

Shapiro, S. L., Brown, K. W., & Biegel, G. M. (2007). Teaching self-care to caregivers: Effects of mindfulness-based stress reduction on the mental health of therapists in training. *Training and Education in Professional Psychology, 1*(2), 105–115.

Shapiro, S. L., Schwartz, G. E., & Bonner, G. (1998). Effects of mindfulness-based stress reduction on medical and premedical students. *Journal of Behavioral Medicine, 21*(6), 581–599.

Srinivasan, M. (2014). *Teach, breathe, learn: Mindfulness in and out of the classroom.* Berkeley, CA: Parallax Press.

Tang, Y. Y., Ma, Y., Wang, J., Fan, Y., Feng, S., Lu, Q., Yu, Q., Sui, D., Rothbart, M. K., Fan, M., & Posner, M. I. (2007). Short-term meditation training improves attention and self-regulation. *Proceedings of the National Academy of Sciences, 104*(43), 17152–17156.

Treasure, J. (2011). *Sound business.* Oxford: Management Books 2000 Limited.

Varona, D. A. (2018). The mindful music educator: Strategies for reducing stress and increasing well-being. *Music Educators Journal, 105*(2), 64–71.

8 Roots

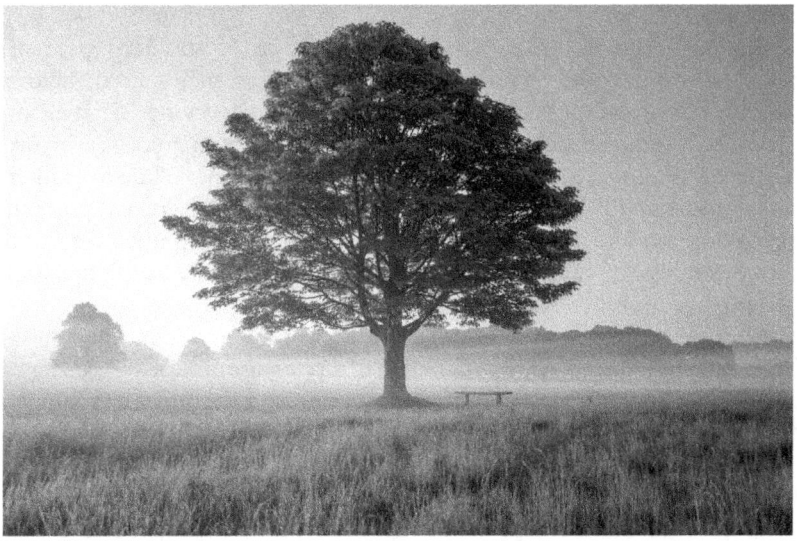

Figure 8.1 Roots
Source: Simon Wilkes, Unsplash, https://unsplash.com/

The process of writing this book has been gratifying, and has provided space to reflect on my own life and career in music education. Thinking about personal experiences with sleep, physical movement, nutrition, gratitude, happiness, and mindfulness has led to the realization that these six variables can indeed be considered as important directional "routes," but also as grounding "roots." Like the cornerstone or foundation of a building, or the growth of a plant or tree, roots are critical support systems to grow and stabilize the beauty of architecture, or branches, bark, and foliage. Happening upon Richard Powers' novel,

The Overstory (2019), during the writing of this book served as an important reminder regarding the roots of both plant and human life.

I was fortunate to grow up in a loving and supportive household, the middle child of a college professor father and devoted homemaker mother in central North Carolina. While there were sometimes challenges, as with all of our lives, the culture was primarily stable and happy. My parents were good about establishing routine sleep schedules, making it clear when my siblings and I needed to be in bed, and patiently encouraging us to sleep longer on those occasional mornings when we woke too early. I vividly remember being allowed to watch *The Love Boat* on Friday nights, but knowing that the following show, *Fantasy Island,* would never be seen, as it was the clear time to brush teeth and get ready for bed.

Similarly, nutritious and regular meals were a standard part of my childhood. Food was always available, and even required, before heading off to school, lunch was prepared in a brown paper bag or purchased in the school cafeteria, and a balanced dinner cooked by my mother was almost always served precisely at 6:00 p.m. While my father was not known for his culinary acumen (he once tried to reheat pizza in a stovetop pan, burning the bottom and leaving the top uncooked), he supported healthy nutrition, regularly joining the family for dinner, and helping our mother to monitor snacking decisions.

Physical movement and exercise were never mandated in our household, but our parents were supportive of opportunities for sports. They enrolled me in youth soccer as a young child, paid for university faculty club membership that provided access to golf, tennis, and swimming, and encouraged me when I started dabbling in light jogging as a teenager. My mother was quite athletic, having participated in team gymnastics and basketball as a youth, and playing competitive tennis well into her adult years. My father walked to work on a daily basis, covering a couple of miles each way, and bragging about his speed per mile (as fast as 12–13 minutes per mile) and annual distance traveled by foot (always well over 1,000 miles).

All of these recollections lead to the deep current feelings of gratitude, and I was taught at an early age to be grateful. Formal opportunities like singing grace before meals or attending weekly Sunday school were clear directives to offer thanks, but my parents and siblings were also strong models of gratitude. Throughout childhood, I was gently guided and often reminded that much of what I took for granted was rooted in privilege. While mindfulness was not a common term at the time, I was introduced to prayer via the Lutheran church, and was encouraged to seek opportunities for solitude and reflection, sometimes through means of required time-outs.

Other forms of positive psychology were also present during my childhood, even though the formal field of study was at best in its infancy. Digital distraction was easy to avoid since personal computers were just coming on the market and the Internet was yet to be. We did have cable television in my early teens, newly offering expanded choices for program viewing. My parents seemed aware of this potential challenge, carefully limiting time spent watching and monitoring the content of shows being viewed. My siblings and I were encouraged to read, and I vividly recall waiting for the afternoon newspaper to arrive after school, just to learn whether my favorite baseball team had won the night before (talk about delayed gratification and development of patience!). Life meaning was also part of regular conversations and goals, particularly as it came time to choose a college major and consider potential life paths. My father, a professor of industrial engineering, was not initially thrilled when I introduced the idea of studying music at college. He was even more surprised when I mentioned the possibility of teaching in K-12 schools. To his credit, he listened to my mother and patiently listened to my reasons for pursuing music education. Realizing that his call to a life of math and quantitative reasoning was similar to the potential life meaning I found in music, my father eventually became excited about the possibility, with my entire family becoming strong supporters and sources of encouragement for the future.

College years provided plenty of opportunities and challenges, but the existing structure helped to keep my practices related to sleep, physical movement, nutrition, and positive psychology relatively under control. I certainly made mistakes, occasionally gorging on chips, cookies, and questionable take-out food, while neglecting healthy sleep and physical movement practices. But I would learn from these lessons, and had the benefit of youth on my side, usually bouncing back from bad health decisions without too much effort. My first year in the teaching profession was a different story.

The initial K-12 teaching position included work at three schools, one elementary, one middle, and one high school, none of which fed each other. To add to the challenge, all three schools involved teaching string orchestra (I had been a horn major, completing a semester of student teaching with middle school band). The final piece of the stress-inducing trifecta was the fact that I was hired just ten days before the new school year started. Not surprisingly, I found little time for sleep, physical movement, or healthy nutrition. While I did enjoy many facets of that first teaching year, I felt like I was constantly struggling to keep up, learning string secondary instruments, meeting new people, and negotiating the ropes of teaching on my own.

Adding to the stress, I lived alone in an apartment near one of the schools, and for the first time in my life, felt like I was lacking in close friendships. My college peers had moved on to other careers and locations, my new colleagues were mostly a generation older, and it was obviously inappropriate to befriend any high school students. Most evenings, I arrived home feeling exhausted and ate inexpensive take-out food. Our high school sold buy-one, get-one-free coupon books for fundraising, and I vividly recall buying one whopper, large fry, and large soda, and receiving another whopper, large fry, and large soda for free! After consuming the entire double meal by myself, there was certainly no energy for exercise, and my mental state suffered.

Slightly healthier choices over the next few years helped, I met a great partner, and eventually left my K-12 position to enroll in doctoral studies. While this was a challenging move, I became engaged to be married during the transition, and my fiancée helped motivate me to eat well and exercise on a regular basis. While I had dabbled in jogging on and off since high school, I became an avid runner during doctoral studies, eventually completing my first full marathon. I also became more aware of research in psychology and musicians' health, even considering a related topic for my dissertation (interestingly, my faculty advisor warned against this idea, stating that such a topic might be too controversial for the profession at that time).

Doctoral studies led to a great job in western New York, but again, the pressure mounted to prove myself in a new environment. To add to that stress, my wife was never very happy about moving several states away, and she was starting to notice her mother slipping into bad health. My mother-in-law quickly developed severe dementia, and the decision was made to move her into our house in New York. While I generally enjoyed work, home life became very difficult, and there was quite a bit of pressure to find a new job in a location closer to our original homes in North Carolina. I spent lots of time and energy applying for and interviewing for many jobs, including a few nice offers. However, I kept coming back to the feeling that what I already had was too good to leave.

Recognition of this gratitude for New York, and the tailwinds in life that were positively combating the headwinds, was very helpful, but it didn't solve all problems. Sleep was difficult and inconsistent, often leading to poor choices with nutrition and non-existent formal exercise. My mood slumped, my wife noticed, and we eventually made the difficult decision to part ways (although we remain friends to this day). Once again alone, I felt a lot like that first year of K-12 teaching. Many colleagues were still a generation older, and it was inappropriate to befriend even graduate students or alumni of our program.

During these first few years in higher education, I also noticed stress and fatigue among our college students and some K-12 music teachers in the area. While combating my own life challenges, I started reading and doing a bit of survey research in the field of music teacher and college student burnout. It was helpful to know that others struggled with similar challenges, and useful to share these findings with students and teachers. Feedback was positive and my career was moving forward nicely. Despite these professional accomplishments, my personal life remained challenging and, to some extent, immersing myself in the pathology of unhealthy individuals only added to my own stress.

After getting away from burnout research for a few years, dabbling in a bit of administrative work and studying the field of improvisation, I still craved information about mental health. As I began reading more literature, I was intrigued to learn about the field of positive psychology. There was very little discussion of this topic at music conferences and in related publications, but academic departments and professional journals were becoming dedicated to the discipline. The past few years have continued in this direction, and in addition to my own research, many other music education researchers are incorporating facets of positive psychology with both PK-12 music teachers and preservice candidates.

Fortunately, my own health has taken a turn for the better, and has ultimately led to motivation for this book. I've found that making positive adjustments to one area of health leads to improvements in other areas. For example, while assessing my own sleep routine, I realized that I was usually around bed and thinking about sleep for seven to eight hours per night, but that I was only sleeping for a little over six hours on a regular basis. By winding down earlier at night and setting a specific time to stop checking email and social media, I've improved actual sleep time to a little over seven hours per night (and often make space for a short afternoon power nap). These adjustments have led to greater morning energy and productivity, and have helped to exercise more and make better food choices. Ultimately, I have a more positive perspective on life, which leads to greater levels of gratitude, happiness, and mindfulness.

A Few Further Recommendations

In addition to the preceding chapter suggestions regarding sleep, physical movement, nutrition, gratitude, happiness, and mindfulness, the following recommendations have helped me to feel greater wellness and vitality, and are all backed by research (e.g., Diener & Biswas-Diener, 2008; Peterson, 2018; Seligman, 2011; Wachob, 2016). Autonomy is the notion that individuals who have the freedom to self-regulate and the ability to act alone are more likely to experience life satisfaction than those who are controlled by others. Yu, Levesque-Bristol, and Maeda (2018) conducted a meta-analysis of 36 studies correlating the need for autonomy and subjective well-being among 12,906 participants from Japan, China, and the United States, and found that autonomy is indeed a universal psychological need. However, Elmore and McPeak (2019) suggested that teachers, parents, and bosses/administrators often stifle the autonomy of those they supervise, unintentionally limiting creativity and growth among students, children, and employees. It is important that music teachers trust their students and create space for learning, while simultaneously being given latitude and respect by their administration. As a respected mentor of mine once said, "hire good people and let them do their job."

Organization and consistency of schedule are both important for life flourishing. Hard copy or digital planners can be used to manage dates and activities, as well as other thoughts that need to be remembered without cluttering mental space. Prevatt et al. (2011) developed a 50-item self-report survey to measure academic and personal variables among college students. They found that higher functioning students tended to report better organization and use of tools such as organizers, planners, calendars, binders, and to-do lists, and recommended that each student set achievement goals for specific courses, and then devise a plan in order to reach each goal. "For example, the student should set specific homework/study times for each week in order to obtain an end of the semester goal" (p. 29). In addition, it's useful to tackle important projects early in the day. Prioritizing tasks that need to happen sooner rather than later allows space to successfully complete expectations on time, pushing more pleasurable activities or things that can wait until later in the day (sometimes being bumped to a later date if necessary). Tracy (2002) presented the concept of "eating that frog," translating to completing essential tasks for a given day as early as possible.

> The purpose of time-management skills, of eating that frog, and getting more done in less time, is to enable you to spend more face time with the people you care about, doing the things that give you the greatest amount of joy in life.
>
> (p. 1)

Similarly, scheduling breaks throughout a given day provides space for relaxation and contemplation. Current society, particularly related to the music education profession, is often obsessed with busyness and productivity. While these can seem like worthy goals, constant activity, in addition to perceptions of others being one step ahead of us, usually leads to feelings of anxiety and fatigue. Creating time to simply be will often help reduce stress and ultimately enhance productivity.

> The people who maintain a happy life, those who are emotionally healthy, are people who create margin in their calendars. They schedule portions of their days to create space. They remove noise and clutter during those portions of time. They experience solitude. Quiet. Simplicity. They take control of their days instead of remaining at the mercy of all the busyness going on. They are intentional to unplug.
> (Elmore & McPeak, 2019, p. 146)

Bono (2020) recommended time to restore following activities involving high energy and extroverted socializing, allowing arousal levels to return to their natural baseline. This can be particularly important for teachers who are naturally introverted. Finding a quiet space and taking even just a few minutes at various points during a school day can provide release of pressure and renewal of energy. Interestingly, Mogilner, Chance, and Norton (2012) found that giving some time to others via generosity can enhance psychological perceptions of overall time. They conducted four experiments in which spending time on other people was compared to wasting time, spending time on oneself, and being given an unexpected long period of free time. "The impact of giving time on feelings of time affluence is driven by a boosted sense of self-efficacy. Consequently, giving time makes people more willing to commit to future engagements despite their busy schedules" (p. 1233).

Play is an important component for all human beings, even adults. Returning to childlike simplicities of life can create energy, enjoyment, and spontaneity. Brown and Vaughan (2010) suggested that play is essential to sound neurological and social development. "In play, most of the time we are able to try out things without threatening our physical or emotional well-being. We are safe precisely because we are just playing" (p. 34). Unfortunately, even children miss out on some of these experiences in the current age of digital attachment and physical inactivity.

> Our focus groups revealed that a large percentage of middle school students derive their senses of identity from social media, which destines them to be on an emotional roller coaster. Millions are restless at night, on a screen instead of sleeping, and restless during the day, always changing in response to circumstances. Eleven percent of Generation Z have been diagnosed with ADHD. As a kid,

> my sense of identity came from my family, my sports team, and where I sat in the lunchroom. Today, it's online.
>
> (Elmore & McPeak, 2019, p. 28)

Higdon (2019) further cautioned that play can be lost in urban and digital spaces, recommending that planners make room for related opportunities in both child and adult populations. Play returns us to a state of sound psychological functioning, reminding us to avoid taking things too seriously and that difficult moments are usually temporary. This, too, shall pass.

Play can also lead to improved self-care. In a culture that celebrates hard work and busyness, taking time to renew and focus on the self is particularly important. Consider required instructions from flight crews during airplane travel. In the unlikely event of cabin pressure loss, be sure to assist yourself with an oxygen mask before helping others. This type of advice is particularly important in the teaching profession. Healthy educators "take care of themselves, intentionally resting, exercising, and relaxing" (Upbility, 2020). A recent undergraduate music education major took pride in what he called, "Self-care Sunday," a regularly planned part of every week when he knew he would slow down to enjoy a good meal, read for pleasure, and do a bit of relaxed yoga. Anderson, Burford, and Emmerton (2016) examined the effectiveness of mobile health apps as monitors for self-care. They performed qualitative analyses of 22 consumers regulating issues such as diabetes, depression, blood pressure, and fitness. While digital applications were helpful to many, the authors found that quality of app and ease of use compromised motivation, and that many participants lost interest in technology after initial use.

Lifelong learning serves as the final recommendation for this book. While that might seem like another arduous task, leading to further stress and burnout, curiosity for new information is a hallmark of the human condition, and when set in an autonomous environment, will often lead to feelings of vigor and enjoyment. Lifelong exploration also ensures that music teachers will continue to embrace the role of learner, bringing new information and fresh perspectives as careers progress. Longworth (2019) argued that continued learning is critical to societal growth in education, business, and government, and suggested that values and attitudes related to lifelong learning are as important as skills and knowledge. Boyatzis, Smith, and Van Oosten (2019) supported this notion, and stated that helping others through a lens of compassion can be particularly helpful.

While change is not always easy, taking gradual steps to implement suggestions from this book can help negotiate routes to wellness and vitality. By implementing sound practices for sleep, physical movement, nutrition, gratitude, happiness, and mindfulness, we can further grow and deepen roots for sustained health. Like the hypothetical characters from preceding chapters, Zach, Rhonda, Tony, Paul, Felicia, and Amy, we can move from sluggish or anxious feelings of stress and burnout to fulfillment and enjoyment of music education. For those feeling out of balance in more than one area of the six main chapters, I encourage you to focus on one issue at a time. As mentioned previously in this chapter, recent changes to my sleep routine have helped other areas. By going to bed a bit earlier than usual, I avoid the temptation of poor nutrition choices late at night, and usually wake up early enough to enjoy a good workout before starting each workday. As a reminder, strong challenges should be addressed with the aid of a licensed medical professional, but small steps can lead to great gains. I wish you all the best on your journey to wellness and vitality in music education.

Summary

- Enjoy sleep, physical movement, nutrition, gratitude, happiness, and mindfulness.
- Strive for autonomy and engender it in others.
- Plan and organize. Create a system for daily structure.
- Prioritize to complete important tasks early in the day.

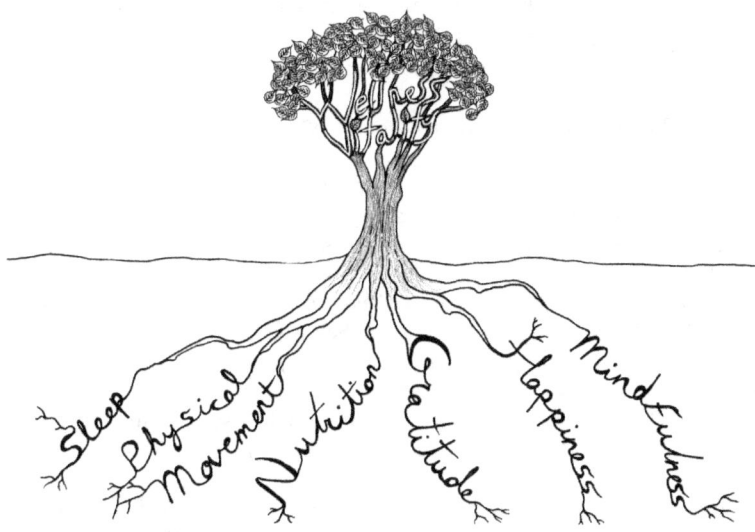

Figure 8.2 Zimmerman Hand Drawing 2
Source: Roots of Wellness and Vitality, Samantha Zimmerman

- Create regular spaces of time to simply be. Avoid unproductive busyness.
- Give to others. Generosity increases perceptions of time.
- Play. Return to the joy and simplicity of childhood.
- Treat yourself. Allow room for some self-indulgence.
- Remain a lifelong learner.

References

Anderson, K., Burford, O., & Emmerton, L. (2016). Mobile health apps to facilitate self-care: A qualitative study of user experiences. *Plos One*. Retrieved February 15, 2020, from https://doi.org/10.1371/journal.pone.0156164

Bono, T. (2020). *Happiness 101: Simple secrets to smart living and well-being*. New York, NY: Grand Central.

Boyatzis, R., Smith, M. L., & Van Oosten, E. (2019). *Helping people change: Coaching with compassion for lifelong learning and growth*. Cambridge, MA: Harvard Business Press.

Brown, S. & Vaughan, C. (2010). *Play: How it shapes the brain, opens the imagination, and invigorates the soul*. New York, NY: Penguin Books.

Diener, E. & Biswas-Diener, R. (2008). *Happiness: Unlocking the mysteries of psychological wealth*. Malden, MA: Blackwell.

Elmore, T. & McPeak, A. (2019). *Generation Z unfiltered: Facing nine hidden challenges of the most anxious population*. Atlanta, GA: Poet Gardener.

Higdon, S. (2019). Taking play seriously: The importance of play and urban play space design. *Cache*. Retrieved from http://hdl.handle.net/10920/36600

Longworth, N. (2019). *Making lifelong learning work*. London: Routledge.

Mogilner, C., Chance, Z., & Norton, M. I. (2012). Giving time gives you time. *Psychological Science, 23*(10), 1233–1238.

Peterson, J. B. (2018). *12 rules for life: An antidote to chaos*. Toronto, ON: Random House Canada.

Powers, R. (2019). *The overstory: A novel*. New York, NY: W. W. Norton & Company.

Prevatt, F., Li, H., Welles, T., Festa-Dreher, D., Yelland, S., & Lee, J. (2011). The academic success inventory for college students: Scale development and practical implications for use with students. *Journal of College Admission, 211*, 26–31.

Seligman, M. E. P. (2011). *Flourish: A visionary new understanding of happiness and well- being*. New York, NY: Simon & Schuster.

Tracy, B. (2002). *Eat that frog: 21 great ways to stop procrastinating and get more done in less time*. San Francisco, CA: Berrett-Koehler.

Upbility. (2020). Retrieved February 25, 2020, from https://www.upbility.net

Wachob, J. (2016). *Wellth: How to build a life, not a résumé*. New York, NY: Harmony Books.

Yu, S., Levesque-Bristol, C., & Maeda, Y. (2018). General need for autonomy and subjective well-being: A meta-analysis of studies in the US and East Asia. *Journal of Happiness Studies, 19*, 1863–1882.

Index

Note: Entries in **bold** denote tables.

acceptance 65
age-related deterioration 4, 23, 28, 30
alcohol 34, 36; and sleep 12–13, 15
Alexander Technique 25–6
American Heart Association 23–6
amygdala 11
anger: and laughter 47; and meditation 69–70
anxiety 4; and attention span 53; and disappointment 46; and gratitude 41; and meditation 70; and mindfulness 64; and physical movement 21; and sleep 14; social media as source of 59
attention, and meditation 69–70
attention span 53, 55
autonomy 57, 79–80
awareness 3–4; and eating 35; and gratitude 44–5; and happiness 56; and mindfulness 64, 66–70

bedtime rituals 14
beginner's mind 65
blessings 42, 45–6
BMI (body mass index) 30
body awareness 22, 69
body posture 59
body scan 65–7, 69, 71
breathing exercises 14–15, 26, 71
breathing meditation 65–6, 69
burnout 1–3; author's research on 79; and personal accomplishment 59
busyness 80–2

caffeine 12, 36
cancer 4; and nutrition 30, 36; and physical movement 20; and sleep 10
carbohydrates 24, 31–4
cataracts 4, 30
catastrophizing 64
cheese 32
coffee 17, 30, 34, 36
cognitive behavioral therapy 3
cognitive functions, and physical movement 21
comparison, interpersonal 57
compassion 69–70, 82
competition, negative aspects of 46–7
constipation 4, 30
contemplation 45
cortisol 21, 70
COVID-19 2
creativity 4, 11, 13, 41, 80
curiosity 4, 64, 66, 82

dairy products 32–3, 36
dehydration 24, 31–2, 36; *see also* hydration
depersonalization 2, 59
depression 4, 52; and gratitude 41–2; and meditation 70; and mindfulness 64; and physical movement 21–2; and sleep 10
diabetes 4, 20, 30–2, 36
diet *see* eating; nutrition
digital devices 14; *see also* smartphones

Index

digital distraction 17, 55, 58, 77
disappointment 46, 60, 64
distance education 2, 47
distress 2–3, 24, 45–6, 53, 70
dopamine 22
doughnuts 33–4

eating: mindful 35, 71; serving sizes 35; and sleep 12, 15; time of day for 34; *see also* nutrition
"eating that frog" 80
endorphins 22
engagement, and happiness 4, 52–6
enjoyment, perceived 23
entitlement, sense of 46, 60
ethical response 42
eustress 2
exercise *see* physical movement
exercise contagion 24
exhaustion, emotional 2, 59

face-to-face interactions 58–9
fatigue 25, 60, 70, 79, 81
fats, dietary 30–4
Feldenkrais Method 25
flourishing 52–3
foam rolling 25
focus: and happiness 57; and physical movement 22
fruits 33–4, 36

gender: and gratitude 42; and physical movement 24
generosity 41, 53, 65, 81
gift-giving 41–2
goal-setting 80
grace before meals 45, 76
grains 31–4, 36
gratitude 3–4, 40–3; author's reflections on 76, 79; and mindfulness 65; recommendations for practicing 44–7
gratitude interventions 44
Gratitude Questionnaire – Six Item Form 43, **43**
grit 60
growth mindset 57
gut microbes 34

happiness 51–4; author's reflections on 79; Bono on 3–4, 46, 52; recommendations for practicing 56–60; studies on 54–6
headwinds 45–6, 78
health: foundations of 4–5; mental 14, 52, 70, 79
heart disease 20, 22, 30, 36
hope 57
hydration 24, 31, 34

identity, sense of 81–2
insomnia 9, 15
isolation 3, 58

journaling 45

Kastor, Deena 42–3

laughing 47
learning, lifelong 82
letting go 65
life satisfaction 4; and gratitude 41, 46; and happiness 54–5, 57
lifestyle changes 4, 10
light, and sleep 13–14, 21
listening: as mindfulness practice 68–9; and physical movement 24
loneliness 47, 58; *see also* isolation

macronutrients 24, 32
materialism 4, 41
MBSR (Mindfulness-Based-Stress-Reduction) 65, 70
MBTI (mindfulness-based therapy for insomnia) 15
meaning: development of 57; and happiness 4, 52–6
meditation 15; apps for 14; in higher education 69–71; for mindful eating 35; moving or walking 22–3; *see also* breathing meditation
melatonin 14
memory loss 4, 30–1
micronutrients 30, 32
milk 32, 34
mindfulness 3–4, 63–5; author's reflections on 76, 79; and eating 35–6; in educational practice 68–71; and physical movement 22, 25; practices of 65–8; and sleep 15

motivation: for physical movement 24; reframing sources of 58
motor skills 11
music, and physical movement 24–5
music education, mindfulness in 68–9
music therapy 3

naps 12
natural foods 36
negative thoughts and emotions 45, 47, 52–3
non-judging 65
non-striving 65
NREM sleep 10, 12–13, 15, 20
nutrition 4, 29–33; author's reflections on 76–9, 83; and physical activity 24; recommendations for healthy 33–7

obesity 20, 30–2
oils, vegetable 32–4, 36
optimism 4, 41
organization 80
Orientation to Happiness 54, **55**
osteoporosis 4, 30

patience 65, 77
personal accomplishment 2, 58–60
personal trainers 24
physical movement 4, 19–20; author's reflections on 76–8; benefits of 13, 21–3; and gratitude 44; and mindfulness 71; and natural light 14; and nutrition 34; recommendations for 23–5; and sleep 13–14; and social interaction 23–4
play 81–2
pleasure 37, 52–5
positive emotions 4, 45, 53, 56–7
positive psychology 3–4; author's reflections on 77; on gratitude 41, 46; and happiness 52–3, 57–8
Powers, Richard 75–6
prayer 42, 76
prioritization 80
privilege, recognition of 45
processed foods 31, 34, 36
productivity 10, 79–81

proteins 24, 31–4
psychological defense systems 53
psychological wealth 52

reflection: and gratitude 45; space for 3
regret, excessive 64
relationships, and happiness 58–9
REM sleep 10, 13, 15, 20
resilience 57
roots 75–6, 83
rumination 15, 64, 70

scheduling, author's reflections on 80–1
school day, beginning of 10
self-care, improved 82
self-confidence 52, 59
self-efficacy 23, 59–60, 81
self-esteem 2, 4, 41, 59
self-regulation 69–70, 80
serotonin 21, 59
sleep 4, 9–11; and alcohol 36; author's reflections on 76–9, 83; biphasic 12; and gratitude 43, 45; and happiness 54–5; and physical movement 20–1; recommendations for sound 11–16; stages of 10–11
sleep environment 13
sleep latency 12–13, 15–16, 20
sleep masks 13
sleep quality 12–14, 21
sleep schedule 11–12
sleeping pills 14–16
smart-apps 14, 58, 82
smartphones 26, 58
smiling 47–8
snacking 30, 34, 36
social media 14, 16, 41, 48, 53, 57–9, 81–2
spirituality 41, 45
state anxiety 21
stress: author's reflections on 78–9; management of 3–4; in music teachers 1–3; and physical movement 13, 21, 23; and sleep 14; use of term 2
stretching 14, 20, 26, 67
stroke 4, 20, 30, 36
sugars 31–4, 36

tai chi 25
tailwinds 45, 78
tea 34
thanksgiving 41, 45–7, 58
time: alone 12; lack of 3, 58; perceptions of 81; for writing 45
time-management 80
trait anxiety 21, 70
treat foods 36–7, 53
trust 65

undoing effect 53

vegetables 33–4, 36
visual aids 57

water *see* hydration
willpower 4, 41

yoga 23, 25
yogurt 32, 34

For Product Safety Concerns and Information please contact our EU representative GPSR@taylorandfrancis.com
Taylor & Francis Verlag GmbH, Kaufingerstraße 24, 80331 München, Germany

www.ingramcontent.com/pod-product-compliance
Lightning Source LLC
Chambersburg PA
CBHW051103230426
43667CB00013B/2431